TAI CHI
CH'UAN *and*
MEDITATION

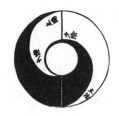

other books by Da Liu:

T'ai Chi Ch'uan and I Ching
The Tao and Chinese Culture
The Tao of Health and Longevity
The Taoist Health Exercise Book

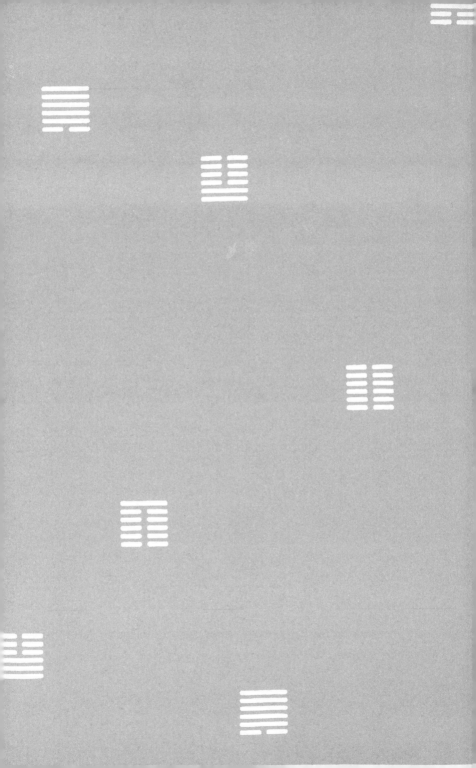

T'AI CHI CH'UAN and MEDITATION

Da Liu

Schocken Books · New York

First published by Schocken Books 1986

Grateful acknowledgment is made to the following for
permission to reprint previously published material:

Crown Publishers, Inc.: Illustration from *Creativity and
Taoism* by Chang Chung-yuan. Copyright © 1963 by Chang
Chung-yuan. Reprinted by permission of Crown Publishers,
Inc.

Thomas Sperling: Illustration of "Yin, Yang" by Thomas
Sperling from *Fundamentals of Yoga* by Rammurti Mishra
(New York: Julian Press, 1971, page 102.) Reprinted by
permission.

Samuel Weiser, Inc.: Photographs from Chu's *Nan: Tao and
Longevity* (York Beach, ME: Samuel Weiser, Inc., 1984.)
Reprinted by permission.

Library of Congress Cataloging-in-Publication Data

Da, Liu.
    T'ai Chi ch'uan and meditation.
Includes index.
1. T'ai chi ch'üan. 2. Meditation (Taoism) I. Title.
GV505.D33   1986   613'.7'1   85-25071
ISBN 0-8052-0993-X

Manufactured in the United States of America
Schocken Books 1991 Edition

19 18 17 16 15

"Who can make the muddy water clear? Let it be still, and it will gradually become clear.

Who can secure the condition of rest? Let movement go on, and the condition of rest will gradually arise."

Tao te ching

To order an instructional videotape containing the complete movements of T'ai Chi Ch'uan found in this book, send a check for $70.00 to Da Liu, T'ai Chi Society of New York, 520 West 110th Street, Apt. 7A, New York, NY 10025.

CONTENTS

PREFACE

In an earlier book, *T'ai Chi Ch'uan and I Ching* (Harper and Row, 1972), I briefly discussed the relationship between T'ai Chi Ch'uan and the practice of meditation. Since the book appeared, I have received many letters from readers interested in this subject. Some have requested a more detailed account of how the T'ai Chi exercises are related to the practice of meditation. Others have expressed doubt and even opposition to the idea of practicing these two disciplines in conjunction with one another. It seems to me that this latter reaction deserves further comment.

Those who object to associating T'ai Chi Ch'uan and meditation are apparently unaware that the T'ai Chi system of exercise was originally developed by the Taoist master Chang San-feng as a form of discipline complementary to meditative practice. More important, they do not recognize that the two disciplines stem from a common source, the *I ching* (*Book of Changes*), and are based on the same yin-yang principle. Although T'ai Chi Ch'uan's character as a system of self-defense is not to be neglected, it is fundamentally a way of becoming in harmony with the basic forces of the universe—the yin and the yang—with the aim of attaining health, longevity, and inner tranquillity. As such, it seeks the same result as meditation, in a complementary way.

I am convinced that in order to obtain the full benefit of the practice of meditation or of T'ai Chi Ch'uan, one must come to understand the philosophical perspective from which they can be clearly seen as two aspects of the same process. As a result, this book contains not merely a practical description of the methods of meditation and exercise, but an explanation of the underlying theory that will enable the reader to practice the techniques in a deeper way. The book may be considered a sequel to and further development of the ideas contained in my earlier book mentioned above. Since that book contained a detailed description of how to perform the T'ai Chi Ch'uan form, that information will not be repeated here. However, I have selected some important movements and related their outer movements to the inner movement of *ch'i* and how this helps meditation.

The sources of the theory that will be explained in this book include not only the *I ching* but also the diagrams known as *T'ai Chi T'u* and the commentaries explaining them written by the neo-Confucian philosophers of the Sung dynasty. These diagrams and commentaries embody the theory more directly and clearly than the *I ching*.

Many Taoist masters have attested to the importance of physical exercise in conjunction with the practice of meditation. Chao Pi Ch'en, the author of *Taoist Yoga* (New York: 1980), a comprehensive exposition of the methods of Taoist meditation, emphasized that the meditator should practice physical exercise to strengthen the body and to help to open the psychic centers important for meditation more effectively than the practice of meditation alone. Other masters have also attested to the effectiveness of a combination of meditation and physical exercise such as T'ai Chi Ch'uan. Among these are the famous Li Ch'ing Yuen, who is said to have lived 250 years (1678–1930), the well-known master Li Shou Ch'ian, who lived to his nineties, and the contemporary master Wang Huai Mien, who still practices and teaches T'ai Chi Ch'uan and meditation at the age of eighty-five.

My own conviction about the relationship between T'ai Chi Ch'uan and meditation comes not from the classics or from the testimony of others, however. This book is not a report of my reading or research. It is a result of my own practice and teaching of these disciplines for the past fifty years. My purpose is to show that, at the highest level, the practice of T'ai Chi Ch'uan aims at the same results as meditation, and to present a detailed, intelligible account of the practical relationship between the two techniques.

ACKNOWLEDGMENTS

I would like to thank the people who helped me to complete this book: Dr. Samuel Johnson, Dr. William Chao, Rosemary Birardi, Steven Berko, C. T. Chang, Dr. Susan Delone, Jorg Dreisorner-Lewis, Sharon Wheeler Hadley, Reggie Jackson, Kao Yu Ying Liu, Paul Knopf, Dr. John Lad, Dr. Margot Lasher, Robert Clark, Jean Matthews, Don Lewis, Carmen Gonzalez Tepalian, Noa Nothmann, Joyce Nawy, and Michal Rovner. This book was written over a period of ten years; the manuscript was rewritten several times. Many whose names are not listed here have helped, and I am grateful to them.

T'AI CHI CH'UAN and MEDITATION

INTRODUCTION

The theory and practice of health exercises and meditation are very old aspects of Chinese culture. Indeed, they apparently originated before the beginning of recorded history, and so accounts of how and by whom they were developed must be regarded as legendary. According to a long-held tradition, Huang Ti, the so-called Yellow Emperor, who began his rule around 2700 B.C., practiced a form of exercise called Tao Yin with the aim of increasing his life span. The word *Tao* means "guide," and *Yin* means "leading." These terms give a hint of how the exercise works: the movements of the limbs guide the circulation of the blood so that the tissues throughout the body can be repaired and cleansed more efficiently. The movements also lead the breath in and out of the lungs, so that more oxygen can be inhaled to nourish and energize the body and the poisons can be exhaled more efficiently. Thus movement is the foundation of a discipline that guides and leads the automatic bodily processes so that they will function in a more beneficial way. Of course, not just any movements will have this effect. It is a remarkable thing about Chinese civilization that the secret of how to achieve this was discovered and understood in prehistoric times.

Essential to the practice of Tao Yin was the way in which the movements of the limbs were combined with the breathing. It is actually this combination that makes the exercise so beneficial for health. Huang Ti's exercises were also known as T'u Na. The word *t'u* means "exhale," and *na* means "inhale."

It is said that Huang Ti once went to the K'ung Tung mountains, where he met the immortal sage Kuang Cheng-tze. This master advised him that in order to preserve life, he should be careful not to thoughtlessly stimulate his passions or stir up his

3

emotions, and should often sit quietly and make his mind more peaceful. By following this advice and practicing his exercises, Huang Ti was able to lead an amazing life. His reign as emperor lasted a hundred years. He had over a hundred wives. Eventually he became an immortal and rode off to heaven on the back of a dragon. When the people saw him riding away, they called out for him to stay, for they loved him so much that they didn't want him to leave. And so, as a final gift to them, Huang Ti dropped down his shoes. A tomb said to contain these shoes still exists in Shanxi Province.

The activities of Huang Ti were precursors of the methods of Taoist meditation and of the form of exercise known as T'ai Chi Ch'uan. These practices did not become widespread during the time of Huang Ti, however. In fact, he is said to have tried to keep them secret. The full development of Taoism did not take place until much later, as we will see in Chapter 1.

The theory behind these practices is based ultimately on the Tao as a joining together of opposites, the fundamental principle of Taoist philosophy. The two opposing manifestations of the Tao, called yin and yang, have universal significance and apply to the phenomena of the cosmos as well as to the operations of the human body. On the largest scale, heaven is yang, while earth is yin. Day is yang, while night is yin. Bright and clear weather is yang; dark and stormy weather is yin. On the scale of living things, the male is yang, the female yin. Spirit is yang, body yin. The opposition applies to the parts of the body and their functions as well. In the circulatory system, the arteries are yang; the veins are yin. In breathing, exhalation is yang; inhalation is yin. In human activities, movement is yang; rest is yin.

A systematic description of the relationships of yin and yang is found in the hexagrams of the *I ching,* the oldest and most important book of Chinese philosophy. The hexagrams themselves date back a couple of centuries before Huang Ti. There is little doubt that his health practices, consisting of an alternation of movement and rest, and his form of exercise involving breathing in and out were direct applications of the yin-yang principle.

This principle has been the basis of the Chinese understanding of health and sickness since ancient times. Good health requires a balance between yin and yang forces within the body. If one or the other is too predominant, sickness results, and it is the aim of the medical sciences, including both acupuncture and herbal medicine, to discover the source of the imbalance and restore the forces to their proper proportion. However, the Taoist philosophy that underlies the practice of T'ai Chi Ch'uan and meditation involves a somewhat more complex theory of the relationship between yin and yang within the body. Taoism does not deny that a general balance between these forces is necessary to avoid sickness. Nevertheless, in a certain respect, it is the aim of meditation to greatly increase the yang and to reduce and diminish the yin. One of the fundamental beliefs of Taoist philosophy is that the reason people become old and weak and eventually die is that they lack sexual energy. This explanation is based on the insight that physical reproduction is but one aspect of the process of maintaining the life and creativity of the individual person. When we are young, our sexual activities naturally generate a powerful energy that pervades all aspects of our life, both physical and mental. The generation of this energy occurs in the production of the sexual essences: the sperm in the male and the menstrual fluid in the female. These substances are both yang. As we grow old and these essences are no longer produced so easily, this natural source of energy tends to dwindle and become less powerful. Thus the sexual essence can be thought of as somewhat like the fuel in a machine. When the machine runs out of fuel, it can no longer move. However, such a loss of energy is not an inevitable result of growing old. Since ancient times, Taoist philosophy has been concerned with the question of how to reproduce and maintain this kind of energy so as to prolong the life and creativity of the individual. The answer to the question is to be found in the methods of Taoist meditation, in which a combination of movement, breathing, and mental concentration is used to purify the sexual essence and distill out its pure yang aspect— that is, pure vital energy—and to transmit it through the eight psychic channels to every cell in the body.

The ultimate aim of such methods, according to the classic Taoist treatises, is nothing short of the attainment of physical immortality. There is no doubt that Taoism has long carried the conviction that this is actually possible. Of course, one would have to be truly exceptional, a person of the stature of Huang Ti, to realize this possibility. Nevertheless, the regular practice of these methods has definitely been shown to result in longevity, good health, vigor, mental alertness, and creativity far beyond what is experienced by most people. In fact, it can also greatly prolong sexual potency and activity, as I will discuss in detail in a later chapter.

In order to obtain the full benefit from this practice, it is essential to understand the principles underlying the methods. Hence it is the aim of this book not only to describe the methods of meditation and exercise, but also to explain how they are based on the philosophy of Taoism. An important insight to be attained through an understanding of this philosophy concerns the way in which the practice of an exercise such as T'ai Chi Ch'uan and meditation should complement one another. The relationship between them manifests a subtle interweaving of opposite (yin and yang) tendencies. This relationship can be seen in the famous diagram known as the T'ai Chi T'u (Diagram of the Supreme Ultimate). This diagram consists of two fishlike figures within a circle: one black, the other white. The black fish, representing rest, is called "greater yin," and the white fish, representing movement, is called "greater yang." Within each figure there is a smaller circle of the opposite color, which may be seen as the eye of the fish. The black circle within the white figure is called "lesser yin" and the white circle within the black figure is called "lesser yang." These inner circles represent the way in which each of the opposing forces, yin and yang, contains within itself its opposite, and also continuously originates from its opposite in a smooth, never-ending cycle. In the practice of T'ai Chi Ch'uan and meditation, the relationship between movement and rest should reflect the interweaving of yang and yin represented in this picture. T'ai Chi Ch'uan, essentially a form of movement, is yang, the white fish. Meditation, which involves standing or sitting quietly, is yin, the black fish. But this distinction takes into account only the external aspects of these activities. To perform the T'ai Chi Ch'uan exercise correctly, one must be very peaceful and quiet inside while executing the externally visible movements. Conversely, the meditator must use the breath and mental concentration to move the vital energy through the psychic channels while remaining externally at rest. Thus the inner aspect of each of these practices is opposite to its outer aspect, just as the greater yang contains the lesser yin within it, and vice versa, as pictured in the diagram.

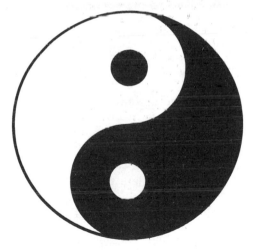

Seen in yet another way, the picture represents the way in which exercise and meditation grow out of one another as alternating practices. The movements of T'ai Chi Ch'uan, while producing more and more energy and vitality, tend to increase the yang side of the yin-yang balance in the body. Eventually, when the yang reaches a high point, it generates a need to sit quietly and purify the energy. This is done through meditation, which produces a more peaceful condition, increasing the yin side of the balance. When the yin reaches a high point, it generates a need to increase the yang once again. Thus it is through the alternate practice of these two opposite methods that one can obtain beneficial effects, including longevity. The achievement of longevity through the alternating cycle of yin and yang activities is thus based on a fundamental principle of Taoist philosophy. Chou Tun-i (1017–1073), the great neo-Confucian philosopher of the Sung dynasty, expressed the principle as follows in his treatise *T'ai chi t'u shuo* (The Diagram of the Supreme Ultimate Explained):

> The Supreme Ultimate through movement produces the yang. This movement, having reached its limit, is followed by quiescence, and by this quiescence it produces the yin. When quiescence has reached its limit, there is a return to movement. Thus movement and quiescence, in alternation, become each the source of the other. The distinction between the yin and yang is determined, and their two forms stand revealed.[1]

This theory of the alternation of yin and yang is coordinated with the principles of T'ai Chi Ch'uan and meditation. After practicing T'ai Chi Ch'uan for a long time, one should rest and practice meditation. Then, after becoming very quiet through meditation, one should practice the movements of T'ai Chi Ch'uan once again to stimulate the blood circulation, release physical stagnation, and relax the mind.

I will discuss the philosophy of Chou Tun-i and of other Taoist scholars in detail in a later chapter, in which it will become clearer what is meant by the two forms of yin and yang. The basic principle is much older than the writings of Chou Tun-i, however. Actually, it is to be found in the *I ching* itself. As the seventeenth-century scholar Wang Ch'uan-shan pointed out, the *I ching* never speaks of "birth and destruction" but only of the alternation of "coming and going."[2] And the text of the *I ching* intimates the same principle in the commentary on hexagram 32, Heng (Duration): "Duration means that which lasts long. The strong is above, the weak below; . . . Gentle and in motion. The strong and the weak all correspond: this signifies duration."[3] The words *strong* and *motion* symbolize the exercise; *weak* and *gentle* symbolize the meditation. Together they bring about duration, that is, longevity.

NOTES

1. Quoted in Fung Yu-lan, *A History of Chinese Philosophy*, trans. Derk Bodde, vol. 2 (Princeton, N.J.: Princeton University Press, 1953), p. 435.
2. See Joseph Needham, *Science and Civilization in China*, vol. 2 (Cambridge: Cambridge University Press, 1956), p. 512.
3. *I ching*, trans. Richard Wilhelm and Cary F. Baynes (Princeton, N.J.: Princeton University Press, 1967), p. 546. All subsequent quotations from the *I ching* are from this edition.

CHAPTER ONE

THE HISTORY OF MEDITATION AND EXERCISE IN CHINA

The practice of meditation began in China in prehistoric times. The underlying principles can be found in the *I ching,* which was written over three thousand years ago—at least two centuries before the legendary rule of Huang Ti. Several hexagrams of the *I ching,* which existed prior to the *I ching,* represent and describe both the practice of meditation and the processes that occur in the body as a result of this practice. One example is hexagram 5, Hsu (Waiting). The Chinese character for this hexagram pictures a person meditating in a sitting position. The text, particularly the Judgment, pertains to the flow of vital energy from one psychic channel to another, a process that occurs during meditation.

5. Hsü/Waiting (Nourishment)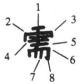

Many of the hexagrams in the *I ching* relate to meditation. Hexagram 5, Hsu, is especially significant. This hexagram symbolizes the process of meditation not only in the Commentary on the Decision, Image, and Lines, but also in the form of the Chinese character itself. Each stroke of the character pic-

tures the form of the meditator: The first stroke symbolizes
the head, the second and third stroke the shoulders and arms,
the fourth and fifth strokes the spinal column and ribs, the
sixth and seventh the bench on which the meditator sits, and
the eighth the legs.

The commentary on the decision gives us the general principle describing the meditation process. "Waiting means holding back" refers to allowing the *ch'i* to mature so that it is
strong enough to rise upward. "Danger lies ahead" warns the
meditator that bad reactions occur when meditation is done
improperly.

However, for those who concentrate and maintain quietness
in meditation, the Commentary says: "If you are sincere, you
have light and success.[1] Perseverance brings good fortune."
Hsu carries a second meaning: Nourishment. This is of special
significance since the Greater Circulation (to be discussed later) of meditation is a process of higher nourishment.

The commentary on the Image for hexagram 5 reveals the
entire process of meditation. "The clouds rise up to heaven"
symbolizes the meditator's energy rising upward as it evaporates into the head, where it is distilled into a salivalike nectar
(referred to in the phrase "the superior man eats and drinks"),
which returns to the abdomen.[2] "It furthers one to cross the
great water" alludes to crossing the great water of the abdomen and mouth.

In addition, each line indicates certain places in the meditator that follow one another. The first line says, "Waiting in the
meadow," which refers to the abdomen, the field of elixir. The
third line, "Waiting in the mud," is the *hui-yin,* or Mortal
Gate, which is the perineum. The fourth line says: "Waiting in
blood. Get out of the pit." Here the *ching* (sexual essence)
turns to *ch'i* (vital energy) as it goes through the *wei-liu,* the
sacrum, also called the Gate of the Tail, and travels up along
the spinal cord toward the head. In the fifth line, "Waiting at
meat and drink" refers to the *ch'i* becoming saliva—what the
Taoists call "the wine of long life." The meditator swallows it
as if he is drinking wine.

The sixth line says: "One falls into the pit," which refers to the saliva going through the throat and down to the *tan-t'ien* (or abdomen). "Three uninvited guests arrive" refers to the three "flowers" that assemble on the top of the head: the *ching* (sexual essence), *ch'i* (vitality), and *shen* (spirit).[3] The sixth line further says: "Honor them, and in the end there will be good fortune." During this time the mediator should keep quiet without being disturbed by the environment and he or she will thus be assured of success.

This completes the process called the Greater Heavenly Circulation for meditation.

Another example the production of saliva and heat in the abdomen is hexagram 63, Chi Chi (After Completion). In this hexagram the upper trigram is K'an (Water) and the lower is Li (Fire). Together they represent the process by which the warmth generated in the abdomen by the concentration of the mind evaporates moisture and sends it upward, resulting in a flow of saliva in the mouth. These insights are not obvious from the *I ching* text, however. As always, the interpretation of the *I ching* is subtle and complex. To explain systematically how the hexagrams are relevant to meditation would require a whole book of its own. The contribution of Huang Ti is easier to understand, since his activities embodied the essential features of movement and breathing in a way that can be directly related to later developments in the techniques of meditation.

LAO TZU

Before considering later developments of techniques, I must mention the philosophy of Lao Tzu. This great master, who lived in the sixth century B.C., was one of the pioneers of the philosophy of Taoism. The principles and viewpoint contained in his famous book, the *Tao te ching,* were deeply influential on all later Taoist thought. Lao Tzu emphasized that "the soft overcomes the hard." Later on many Taoists developed these ideas into Tai Ch'i Ch'uan and meditation.

Chapter 10 of the *Tao te ching* is concerned fundamentally with meditation, but its ideas also relate to the principles of T'ai Chi Ch'uan. If you try to read this chapter literally, it seems illogical; however, Lao Tzu is speaking metaphorically:

Can you keep the spirit and body without scattering?
Can you concentrate your mind to use breath, making it soft and quiet as an infant's?
Can you purify your contemplation and keep it from turbulence?
Can you love the people and rule the state by nonaction?
The gate of heaven opens and closes. Can you be like the female?
Can you become enlightened and penetrate everywhere without knowledge? . . .*

"Can you keep the spirit and body without scattering?" This is the fundamental idea of Taoist meditation. The Taoists believed the body and mind should be united to achieve longevity and immortality.

"Can you concentrate your mind to use breath, making it soft and quiet as an infant's?" The "breath" here is not just ordinary breath. First it must become inner energy.[4] Chuang Tzu says that the respiration of ordinary people is from their throat, and further, that the true men of old breathed from their heels. Infancy is the state in which the body is soft and pliant, and the mind quiet and innocent. The image of the infant further refers to the "holy fetus," which matures in meditation to emerge as the spirit-infant. This is also a fundamental principle of T'ai Chi Ch'uan.

"Can you purify your contemplation and keep it free from turbulence?" When one meditates, millions of thoughts sprout which should be avoided. This turbulence must be cleaned like

---

*One can find many different translations of the *Tao te ching*. As the *I ching* states, "The kind man discovers it and calls it kind; the wise man discovers it and calls it wise; the common people use it every day and are not aware of it." I offer a translation and further interpretation of the passage above in Chapter 12, on sexual energy.

the mirror that must be completely wiped free from dust in order to reflect purely.

"Can you love the people and rule the state by nonaction?" In the Chin dynasty (fourth century), the famous Taoist and alchemist Ko Hung wrote a book, *Po pu tze,* in which he stated: "One's body is like the state, the spirit [mind] like the king, the blood like the officers, and the *ch'i* like the people." Most Taoists have used this metaphor of people and state to describe the body and *ch'i.* Chapter 57 of the *Tao te ching* explains the concept of nonaction as follows:

> Inasmuch as I betake myself to nonaction, the
>   people of themselves become developed.
> Inasmuch as I love quietude, the people of them-
>   selves become righteous.
> Inasmuch as I make no fuss, the people of them-
>   selves become wealthy.
> Inasmuch as I am free from desire, the people of
>   themselves remain simple.

"The gate of heaven opens and closes. Can you be like the female?" This line from Chapter 10 refers to the highest goal of Taoist meditation. When the "holy fetus" matures enough, it is born from the top of the skull, *(ni-wan).*[5]

"Can you become enlightened and penetrate everywhere without knowledge?" This is what Chuang Tzu means when he calls meditation "Sitting and forgetting": "One lets the body drop and drives out hearing and seeing. One avoids shapes and know-hows. It is like a grand penetration."[6]

Chapter 16 of the *Tao te ching* states that "to attain the goal of absolute vacuity, keep to the state of perfect peace. All things come into existence, and thence we see them return. Look at the things that have been flourishing; each goes back to its origin. Going back to the origin is called peace; it means reversion to destiny." This is the principle of meditation. These are only the principles, not the details. Two centuries later, Chuang Tzu made them clearer.

CHUANG TZU

After Lao Tzu, the second great master of Taoism was Chuang Tzu. His writings, although not strictly commentaries on the *Tao te ching,* are entirely consistent with Lao Tzu's ideas and express them in an expanded and generally clearer way.

The application of Chuang Tzu's remarks to the theory of exercise and meditation is not always easy or straightforward. Many readers, and even some translators, have missed the significance of key passages by treating them as vague and metaphysical. One such passage can be found in the chapter entitled *Ta tsung shih* ("The Greatest and Most Honored Master"): "The breathing of the true man came deep and silently. The breathing of the true man comes from his heels, while men generally breathe only from their throats."[7] Many people, refusing to believe that the body can actually breathe through the heels, read this as a metaphor for some metaphysical idea. When it is considered in relation to the beginning of the T'ai Chi Ch'uan form, however, the remark has a clear sense. At the beginning of the form, one stands with feet firmly on the ground, directly below the shoulders. As one begins to inhale, the arms rise and the knees straighten. The effect of this is to lift the vital energy from the toes through the heels up through the legs and then farther upward through the trunk of the body. During the subsequent exhalation, the arms press downward and the knees bend, resulting in a lowering of the vital energy through the body, the legs, and down to the heels again. The point is that in the practice of exercise and meditation, "breathing" refers not only to the movement of air in and out of the lungs, but to a process involving the whole body, including the circulation of oxygen to the extremities through the blood.

Chuang Tzu speaks of this flow of vital energy through the body in other passages as well. In the chapter entitled *Yang sheng chu* ("Principles of Health and Longevity") we find the following advice: "Use your mind to carry the vital energy along your Tu Mo upward constantly. This can keep your body healthy and your life long." This remark has been difficult for translators who have not understood the Taoist principle involved. Gia-Fu Feng and James Legge use the vague phrase "the middle way" (see Chuang Tzu, the Inner Chapters, p. 53).[8] Actually the Tu Mo has a very precise significance as one of the eight psychic channels through which the vital energy flows. It is called the Channel of Control and runs along the back from the coccyx at the base of the spine to the top of the head.

T'ai Chi Ch'uan was not actually developed until centuries after Chuang Tzu. There is clear eidence, however, that Chuang Tzu was aware of methods of exercise coordinated with breathing that were commonly practiced during his time and that may be considered ancestors of the T'ai Chi Ch'uan system. A passage in the chapter entitled *Ko-i* ("Ingrained Ideas") describes the activities of those who nourish the body and desire longevity. Such people spend their time "inhaling and exhaling the breath, expelling the old breath and taking in new," and move "like the sleeping bear" and "stretch and twist the neck like a bird."[9] This passage indicates that the attainment of longevity (and health) requires both breathing exercises and bodily movement. The bear and the bird evidently refer to movements from exercises well known to Chuang Tzu. It was common for exercise methods to include movements adapted from those of animals and birds. There are several examples of this in the T'ai Chi Ch'uan form, which includes movements such as Bring Tiger to the Mountain, Snake Creeps Down, Step Back and Repulse Monkey, White Crane Spreads Wings, and Golden Cock on One Leg. Other animals are mentioned in the *Classics of T'ai Chi Ch'uan* by Wang Tsung-yueh, which speaks of moving like a cat, for example. The function of these movements is to help guide the breathing and the circulation so that the vital energy can flow through the body and have its beneficial effects. Chuang Tzu goes on to speak of those who attain to longevity with the management (of the breath); who forget all things and yet possess all things; whose placidity is unlimited, while all things to be valued attend them:—such men pursue the way of heaven and earth, and display the characteristics of the sages. Hence it is said, "Placidity, indifference, silence, quietude, absolute vacancy, and non-action:—these are the qualities which maintain the level of heaven and earth and are the substance of the Tao and its characteristics."... In his stillness his virtue is the same as that of the Yin, and in movement his diffusiveness is like that of the Yang.[10]

If the movement represents T'ai Chi Ch'uan and the stillness represents meditation, therefore, practicing them together is more efficient for the achievement of longevity. In another passage, he writes about Confucius' student Yen Hui, who speaks of "sitting and forgetting" as a way of freeing one's self from the body and mind and becoming one with the infinite.[11] This passage makes it clear that Chuang Tzu considered meditation to be a way of attaining a state of quietude and emptiness by following the Taoist idea of nonaction and nonbeing.

Chuang Tzu describes two men in the State of Lu. Shan Pao lived among the rocks and drank only water. Until he was seventy, he had still the complexion of a child. Unfortunately he was killed and eaten by a tiger. There was also a Chang I, who worked for the other people. In his fortieth year he fell ill of a fever and died. Of these two men, Shan Pao nourished his inner man and a tiger ate his outer, while Chang I nourished outer man and disease attacked his inner. Both of them neglected "whipping up their lagging sheep." Chuang Tzu means that man should practice meditation and exercise together.

Chuang Tzu lived during the Warring States Period, which continued until 221 B.C., after a short time of unification by the Ch'in dynasty, when the Ch'in dynasty was overthrown. The next four centuries, during which China was ruled by the Han dynasty, were a time of peace as well as creativity in science and the arts. It was during the Eastern Han period (so called because the capital was in the eastern provinces during that time) that the great philosopher Wei Po-yang wrote his fundamental and important book entitled *Ts'an tung ch'i,* which may be translated "The Kinship of the Three, or the Accordance of the *Book of Changes* with the Phenomena of Composite Things." This book develops a method of meditation based on the *I ching,* and also contains much information pertaining to alchemy and its uses. Wei related the idea of the vital energy (*ch'i*) circulating through the psychic channels to the fundamental forces governing the universe on the largest scale. Thus he described the processes of meditation in terms of the philosophy of yin and yang, the five elements, and the waxing and waning of Ch'ien (Heaven) and K'un (Earth). His idea that processes in the body reflect the same principles at work in the cosmos at large had great influence on all later thinking on the theory of meditation. A similar idea was emphasized by another philosopher of the Han period, Liu An, in his famous book *Huai-nan Tzu.*

Some passages in Wei's work suggest that he considered it important to practice exercise in conjunction with meditation. For example, in one chapter he says, "You build a wall around the city so that the people will be safe." The meaning of this remark is not obvious on the surface, but with proper interpretation, it is possible to understand the metaphor. The idea of building a wall around a city (a practice common in ancient times both in China and the West) represents the use of exercise to make the body strong and healthy outside and to prevent sickness. The idea that the people will be safe represents the peacefulness of the mind inside a healthy body that allows the spirit to be active and able to achieve the concentration necessary for the successful practice of meditation.

In the third century A.D. an exercise called the Movement of the Five Animals was invented by Hua T'o, a surgeon. He contributed additional movements of animals such as the bear, tiger, monkey, deer, and bird to the development of T'ai Chi Ch'uan. A series of eighteen forms of health exercise invented by the alchemist Ko Hung (active A.D. 325), completed the evolution of the Tao Yin. This work was discovered on a silk painting in an ancient tomb in Hunan Province in 1974. Ko's system is only for health, not for self-defense.

An important event that took place during the Han dynasty was the introduction of Buddhism into China. By the sixth century A.D., the Buddhist religion had an importance equal to that of Taoism and Confucianism in the Chinese religious and philosophical tradition. Buddhism had a direct influence on the development of meditation in China, for it had its own traditional methods of meditation, which had originated in India independently of the growth of similar methods in China. Buddhists advocated the attainment of peace and tranquility through giving up desire and ridding oneself of the limited personal ego. As a means toward these ends the Buddhists employed meditation.

A particularly important development in the Buddhist meditation tradition was the invention of the Shao Lin method of exercise. This was accomplished by the master Ta Mo (also known as Daruma), who came to China from India around A.D. 530 and established a school of Zen Buddhism in a monastery known as Shao Lin. While teaching meditation and Zen concepts to the monks, he became aware that his students were growing physically weaker. Their bodies were becoming as thin as dry wood, their faces turned pale, and many were sick. Ta Mo thought a great deal about how to restore their health. According to tradition, he sat in meditation facing a wall for nine years. The solution he finally discovered exemplified the fundamental principle of philosophy that out of quietude grows movement. He developed a simple form of exercise to stimulate circulation, loosen the joints, and restore vitality. The monks soon found that regular practice of this exercise enabled them to meditate for long periods without undesirable physical effects.

Later on, Ta Mo and his followers made the exercises more strenuous and systematic, and also developed methods of boxing and using weapons such as knives and sticks. Thus the Shao Lin exercises became a system of martial arts.

Several hundred years later, there was a similar development in the Taoist meditation tradition. The great Taoist master Chang San-feng, who was knowledgeable about all the ancient forms of wisdom, including the *I ching,* Confucianism, Buddhism, and Taoism, created, after a long period of meditation, the system of exercise known as T'ai Chi Ch'uan. His aim was similar to that of Ta Mo: to develop a form of discipline complementary to the practice of meditation, which would also promote health. The resulting exercise method (also called the Wu Tang school, after Wu Tang Mountain in Hubei Province where Chang taught) is different from Shao Lin and has quite distinct results. The movements of Shao Lin are generally strenuous and sometimes very quick. Regular practice of these forms results in the strengthening of the limbs and an increase in the size of the muscles. In T'ai Chi Ch'uan, on the other hand, the movements are done slowly, gently, and evenly from beginning to end, each posture unfolding with the same continuous rhythm. The result is an improvement in circulation and respiration and a strengthening of the internal organs, but no increase in muscles. Because of this contrast, T'ai Chi Ch'uan is sometimes called the Inner School and Shao Lin the Outer School. In spite of these differences, both schools are, at their highest levels, forms of spiritual discipline, and both were originally developed to aid in the practice of meditation.

Eventually, the Shao Lin and T'ai Chi Ch'uan exercises became known throughout China as a result of many displays of self-defense skill by those who had become expert in their practice. Unfortunately, this led people to forget that the exercises were meant to be an aid in the practice of meditation. Many laymen who were interested in self-defense came from far and wide to learn the exercises. Some wanted to use them for revenge. Others wanted to use them for military purposes. Still others wanted to create their own schools of martial arts or to teach the exercises in order to make a living. Very few of these people had the patience or the singleness of mind necessary to learn meditation. In spite of this, the Buddhist and Taoist masters taught the exercises to many laymen, and they in turn taught other people for generation after generation. Before long, there were many different schools and styles of self-defense exercise, but most of those who practiced them were unaware of the relationship between exercise and meditation. This situation continues even today.

Nevertheless, there is continuing evidence that meditation and exercise are each indispensable to the successful practice of the other. This is shown in the benefits of health, vigor, and longevity enjoyed by those who consciously practice both disciplines. It has also been shown in the experiences of masters who have found that, at the highest level, the two blend together automatically and unconsciously.

The famous master Yin Shih Tzu died only a few years ago in China. He was enlightened in both Buddhist and Taoist meditation, which he had practiced for many years. He wrote a book about his experiences, entitled *Yin Shi Tzu's Experimental Meditation for the Promotion of Health,* part of which has been translated into English by Lu K'uan Yu in his book *Secrets of Chinese Meditation.* In it he reported that after he had meditated for many years, concentrating on the opening of the eight psychic channels to allow the energy to flow through them, he achieved a state in which, feeling weightless and very warm, he suddenly began to notice that his body was performing the movements of the exercise quite unconsciously and involuntarily. He wrote:

> These involuntary circular movements were really wonderful and inconceivable. When it [a feeling of vibration] reached the fingers and toes, the latter stretched out to move while the legs bent and straightened alternately.... All these movements to the left and right were natural with the same number of turns in each direction.... After that it moved to my limbs so that my arms swung in quick circles to the left and right while my legs bent and straightened and first the toes and then the heel of one foot kept striking those of the other....[12]

A contemporary Zen master, Huai-chin Nan, also made a deep study of Taoism. He suggests using meditation and exercise together: "After sufficient sleep, with vitality renewed, [one] should then meditate again. If he finds, however, that there is no fatigue in mind or body, it is better to get up to do a little exercise. The spirit thus roused, he will be able to maintain an appropriate and stable state of quietude."[13] Professor Nan mentions in his book that it is helpful for meditation to perform Ch'i Kung (Chinese exercise) and Yoga beforehand. Also after meditation, one can use light exercise. T'ai Chi Ch'uan is a moderate and soft exercise that combines well with meditation.

NOTES

1. "Whenever the practitioner walks, stands, sits, or reclines, he sees a white light in front of him, and, as time passes, this white light changes into a golden one." Lu Ku'an Yu, *Taoist Yoga, Alchemy and Immortality* (New York: Weiser, 1970), p. 60.
2. Lui Yen, an immortal of the Tang dynasty, said in his one-hundred-characters tablet: "The white cloud rises up to the head; honeydew falls."
3. Lu Ku'an Yu, *Taoist Yoga*, p. 74.
4. See William Chao, *The Principle of Life Energy* (Taipei: Chao, 1985).
5. For more on the birth of the holy fetus, see Richard Wilhelm, trans., *The Secret of the Golden Flower,* commentary by C. G. Jung (New York: Harcourt Brace Jovanovich, 1962), and Lu K'uan Yu, *Taoist Yoga.*
6. *The Texts of Taoism,* vol. 1, trans. James Legge (New York: Dover Publications, 1962), pp. 256–57.
7. Ibid., p. 238.
8. Ibid., p. 198.
9. Ibid., p. 364.
10. Ibid., p. 257.
11. Ibid., p. 364.
12. Lu K'uan Yu, *The Secrets of Chinese Meditation* (New York: Weiser, 1964), p. 197.
13. Huai-chin Nan, *Tao and Longevity* (New York: Weiser, 1984), p. 8.

CHAPTER TWO

T'AI CHI T'U: DIAGRAM OF THE SUPREME ULTIMATE

In their efforts to symbolize and describe the continuous opposition and interaction between the fundamental forces of yin and yang in the universe, the great Chinese philosophers of antiquity developed several charts and diagrams whose components represented the various aspects of this relationship. Although a number of different diagrams were created, all were known by the identical name: T'ai Chi T'u. This name has been translated differently into English by various scholars. Joseph Needham uses the term "Diagram of the Supreme Pole." Fung Yu-lan prefers "Diagram of the Supreme Ultimate." Richard Wilhelm suggests "Symbol of the Great Primal Beginning." But since none of these is very clear, I will simply use the Chinese name here.

The T'ai Chi T'u has very broad cultural significance and meaning. Such diagrams occur in profound treatises as part of the explanation of the large-scale processes of the universe, in which the light and dark areas specifically represent heaven and earth. On the other hand, they can also often be seen decorating children's clothes, where they are believed to bring fortune and chase away evil and sickness. The diagrams are especially significant for those practicing Taoism as a religion, and are often found placed in temples and worn on clothing indicating religious observance. These practices have their basis in the *I ching,* in Chapter 5 of the *Ta chuan* (The Great Treatise) where one reads: "That which lets now the dark, now the light appear is Tao." The concept of Tao is both sacred and mysterious. It is one of the central religious notions of the East, not only in China, but also in other East Asian countries including Japan, Indochina, and Korea. A T'ai Chi T'u even appears on the Korean flag, indicating that the concept has political as well as religious connotations there.

Today this current has reached the West, where many books refer to the T'ai Chi T'u, both within the text and as part of the cover design. This symbol may also be recognized on jewelry, medals, buttons, and shirts. In short, the influence of this design by now has spread throughout the world.

THE EVOLUTION OF THE T'AI CHI T'U

A tradition has it that the T'ai Chi T'u originated in prehistory and that even in ancient times people used a round symbol with a light upper half, representing heaven, and dark lower half, representing earth. The entire symbol represents the human being, who is a union of both light and dark. Although there may be some validity in this tradition, it is not supported by clear historical or archaeological evidence. In any case, the oldest written expression of the principle underlying these diagrams is available in the *I ching,* in Chapter 11 of the *Ta chuan:* "There is in the Changes the Great Primal Beginning [T'ai Chi]. This generates the two primary forces. The two primary forces generate the four images. The four images generate the eight trigrams." The *I ching* itself contains no T'ai Chi T'u diagram, but the relevance of this quoted passage for the diagrams will become clear in the following explanation.

According to several scholars of Chinese cultural history, the term *t'ai chi* originally referred to the ridgepole of a house, the horizontal beam at the very top of the roof where the two slanted parts of the roof meet. This topmost pole divides the roof into two parts that face in opposite directions. Because of the direction from which the sun shines on the house, one side is brighter, representing yang, while the other side is darker, representing yin. Naturally, this is constantly in flux as the sun moves across the sky. The side facing the rising sun, which is initially strongly yang in the morning, gradually dims as the sun arcs, while the other side, strongly yin in the morning, gradually brightens until the relationship is reversed by evening. Only at a single moment, perhaps at high noon, are the two sides of the roof equally bright. Thus the roof of the house divided by its ridgepole can be regarded as a symbol of the eternal cycle of alternation that continuously occurs between the two fundamental forces of yin and yang.

By the time of the Sung dynasty (A.D. 960–1279) complex diagrams were developed, and extensive commentaries were written to explain their meaning. Of particular importance was the diagram and commentary entitled *T'ai chi t'u shuo* (Diagram of the Supreme Ultimate Explained) composed by Chou Tun-i, the great neo-Confucian philosopher mentioned earlier in the introduction. Chou explains how the diagram symbolized the production and evolution of all things. (See illustration.) The empty circle at the top represents the Supreme Ultimate (*t'ai chi*), which generates the yang through movement and the yin through quiescence. The circle below it, with its inner crescents of alternating black and white, represents the opposition and interaction between yin and yang. Notice that the yang side contains yin within it and the yin side contains yang within it, just as in the T'ai Chi T'u. Below this circle there is a pattern that contains five smaller circles symbolizing the five elements, which come into being through the interaction between yin and yang. As Chou explains:

> By the transformations of the yang, and the union therewith of the yin, water, fire, wood, metal, and earth are produced. These five elements become diffused in harmonious order, and the four seasons proceed in their course.
> The Five Elements are the one yin and yang: the yin and

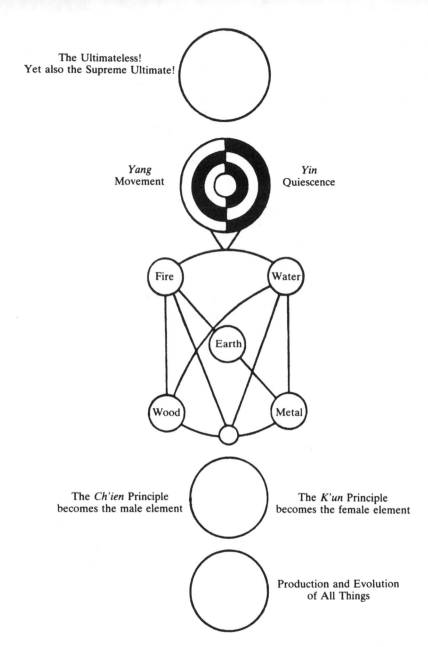

The T'ai Chi T'u of Chou Tun-i
Diagram of the Supreme Ultimate

SOURCE: Fung Yu-lan, *A History of Chinese Philosophy,* vol. 2 (Princeton, N.J.: Princeton University Press, 1953), p. 436.

yang are the one Supreme Ultimate: and the Supreme Ultimate is fundamentally the Ultimateless. The Five Elements come into being each having its own particular nature.[1]

The large circle below the five small ones represents the male and the female joined. Thus the five elements are formed from the yin and yang once again. The lowest circle represents the results of the union of female and male (yin and yang): reproduction of the next generation in the realm of man and in the universe, the production and evolution of all things.

Later Taoists followed the idea of the commentary and the diagram to create T'ai Chi Ch'uan as below. This diagram is closely related to T'ai Chi Ch'uan. Wang Tsung-yueh in his *Classics of T'ai Chi Ch'uan* says: "T'ai Chi (Supreme Ultimate) evolves from Wu Chi (Ultimateless); it is the mother of Yin and Yang. In motion they separate, in stillness they are united."[2]

The uppermost circle symbolizes emptiness—*wu chi*. In the beginning the T'ai Chi Ch'uan player stands quietly with his mind empty. The movements of T'ai Chi Ch'uan correspond to the alternating black and white stripes of the second circle of the diagram. Downward and retreating movements represent the yin, while upward and forward movements represent the yang. The five elements in the five small circles below correspond to the five foot movements performed by the T'ai Chi Ch'uan player, while the eight trigrams of the *I ching* represent the eight movements of the player's hands.* The straight and diagonal connecting lines between the five small circles are an indication of the continuous alternation of the player's steps. Finally, the bottom circle corresponds to the end of the T'ai Chi Ch'uan—a return to stillness.

---

* The five foot movements: Advance, Retreat, Look to Left, to Right, and Central Equilibrium. These five steps equate to the five elements: metal, wood, fire, water, and earth. The eight Movements of Hand: Push up, Pull back, Press forward, Push forward, Pull down, Split, Elbow and Shoulder-strike.

T'AI CHI T'U RELATED TO MEDITATION

Sometime after the death of Chou Tun-i, several scholars discovered that certain sacred books of Taoism that had been written long before Chou's time already contained diagrams very similar to the one he had composed. The most important of these diagrams is the one attributed to the great Taoist philosopher and mathematician Ch'en T'uan (c. 906–989). (See illustration.) Reliable Chinese historians of the seventeenth century report that:

> Ch'en Tuan, while living on the famous "sacred mountain" of Hua Shan in Shensi, had this diagram carved on the face of a cliff. This, they say, consisted of several successive tiers arranged as follows: (1) At the bottom a circle labeled "Doorway of the Mysterious Female." (2) Above this another circle, inscribed: "Transmuting the Essence so as to Transform It into the Vital Force; Transmuting the Vital Force so as to Transform It into the Spirit." (3) The next and central portion represented the elements wood and fire on the left side, metal and water on the right, and earth in the center, all interconnected by lines. It bore the title: "The Five Forces Assembled at the Source." (4) Above this was a circle (or probably several concentric circles), made up of interlocking black and white bands, and entitled: "Taking from *K'an* [water] to Supplement *Li* [fire]." (5) A topmost circle with the inscription: "Transmuting the Spirit so that It May Revert to Vacuity; Reversion and Return to the Ultimateless."[3]

The above clearly refers to meditation also. Ch'en Tuan was an enlightened Taoist and *I ching* philosopher. He adopted Fu Hsi's idea that to create the School of Symbol and Number was an important historical link between traditional and formalized Chinese philosophy and science. He adopted Fu Hsi's Primal Arrangement to create the Taoist T'ai Chi T'u (see illustration) for Taoist meditation. Fu Hsi was the creator of the eight trigrams of the *I ching*.

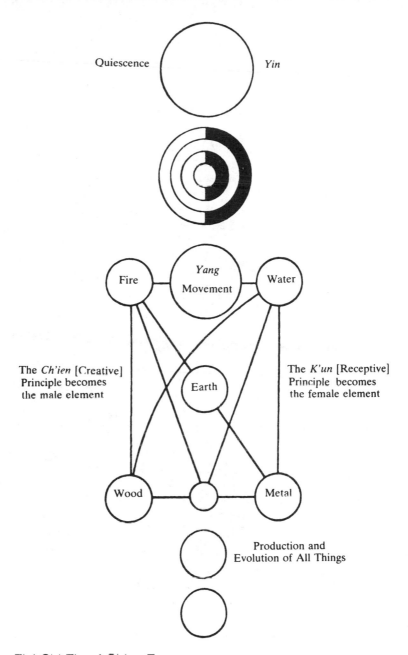

The T'ai Chi T'u of Ch'en Tuan
Diagram of the Supreme Ultimate That Antedates Heaven

SOURCE: Fung Yu-lan, *A History of Chinese Philosophy*, vol. 2, p. 439.

THE "DOUBLE FISH" SYMBOL

The most famous T'ai Chi T'u is the circle containing the "double fish," which I discussed in the Introduction. Others have also had great influence on Chinese thought, however, and will be described below. All these diagrams are similar in that they consist of patterns of black and white, the black areas representing yin and the white areas representing yang.

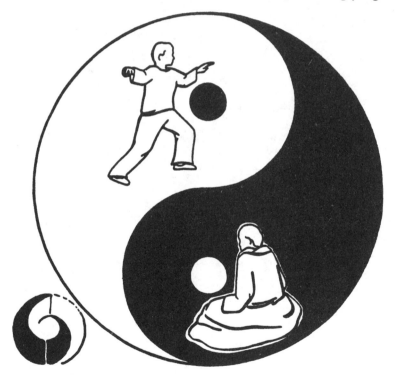

The Double Fish: Symbol of T'ai Chi Ch'uan and Meditation

The double fish is the T'ai Chi symbol. The white fish has a black dot or eye; that means that yang contains yin within it. This symbolizes T'ai Chi Ch'uan, in which the body moves outside but the mind is at peace. The black fish represents yin, quiet, and meditation, while the yang dot or eye symbolizes movement. Meditation is not empty; the mind is used to conduct the breath moving inside. The parts of the Yin-Yang diagram are put together to represent the shape of the universal.

This illustration shows T'ai Chi Ch'uan and meditation united in one symbol. From this symbol I adopted the idea and put the two exercises together in one book—T'ai Chi Ch'uan and meditation.

The illustration of the Lesser Heavenly Circulation is similar to the double fish symbol (see page 32) except that the black dot in the white area becomes a black line and the white dot in the black area becomes a white line. The illustration shows the comingling of "postnatal" and "prenatal" breathing, which occur in Taoist deep breathing technique. The white circle in the center represents the navel. The black line extending from the top of the large circle to the navel represents postnatal (regular) breathing. The white line below represents prenatal (fetal) breathing. In regular breathing oxygen is inhaled and drawn down into the navel. At the same time, fetal breathing is drawn up into the navel. The regular breath is returned through exhalation to the outside, and the fetal breath is returned to the lower abdomen.

The circulation of oxygen and fetal breath is referred to as the union of K'an (Water) and Li (Fire). The trigram K'an, shown at the bottom of the white line, consists of two yin lines outside and one yang line inside. White is the color of yang. Therefore the white line represents K'an, or prenatal (fetal) breath. The trigram Li, shown at the top of the black line, consists of two yang lines outside and one yin line inside. Black is the color of yin, and therefore the black line represents Li, or postnatal breathing. This union of Kan and Li is also called the Lesser Heavenly Circulation.

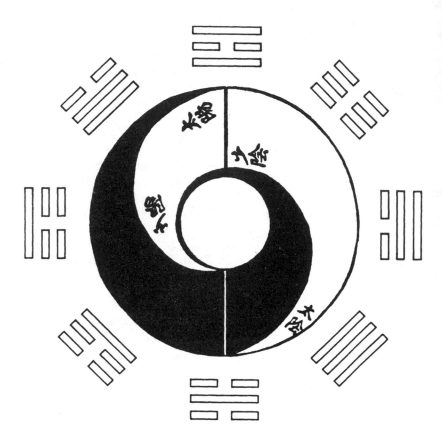

The Lesser Heavenly Circulation

The most advanced practitioners of Taoist meditation and T'ai Chi Ch'uan are able to use the prenatal breathing technique. It is only when the practitioner has attained a certain level that the breathing can reach the navel and draw up the prenatal breath into the same region.

NOTES

1. Quoted in Fung Yu-lan, *A History of Chinese Philosophy*, vol. 2, p. 437.
2. Ibid.
3. The historians Huang Tsung-yen (1616–1686) and Chu Yi-tsun (1629–1709) are quoted in Fung Yu-lan, p. 441.

CHAPTER THREE

FUNDAMENTALS OF CHINESE PHYSIOLOGY

In order to learn the Taoist disciplines of meditation and exercise successfully, it is important to know the basic concepts of Chinese physiology. This requirement is analogous to the Western idea that one cannot easily develop athletic skills without being aware of the processes going on in the body through the study of anatomy and physiology. Both meditation and related forms of exercise such as T'ai Chi Ch'uan involve the circulation of energy throughout the body. To experience this circulation, one needs to have a precise notion of the location of specific points and the pathways or channels between these points along which the energy flows.

The traditional Chinese concept of the human body differs somewhat from the Western one. The most important difference is that Chinese physiological descriptions make use of terms and ideas that Westerners regard as spiritual or psychic. For example, *ch'i,* or vital energy, does not refer to any physical entity that can be detected or measured with scientific instruments. It is an invisible psychic substance that can only be felt inside the body as it flows through the psychic channels. The five points, the eight psychic channels, and the twelve meridians that run along the surface of the body are likewise invisible and cannot be detected by physical methods. The Western scientific mind, which tends to view the body as a chemical machine, is likely to regard such psychic concepts with considerable skepticism. They have great importance in Chinese thought, however, for they are not only essential in the theory of meditation, but also form the basis of the theory underlying a very advanced and highly sophisticated medical technology, including acupuncture and acupressure. (Incidentally, the Chinese are not the only culture to have developed such concepts in investigating the human body. The Indian Yoga tradition uses similar ideas, although the terminology employed is quite different. The other Eastern martial arts—Japanese Aikido and Judo, Korean Ta Kuan Tao and Viet Boxing—also make use of meditation as a means of achieving the highest level of skill.)

THE EIGHT PSYCHIC CHANNELS

Eight connective pathways that both transmit and store energy are located in the trunk of the body and in the arms and legs. Through them, energy can reach every cell in the body. The method of systematically circulating the *ch'i* through all of these channels during meditation was proved effective and definitively described by the famous Taoist master Yin Shih Tzu, who died only recently, in his treatises on the methods of meditation.[1] The names and locations of the eight psychic channels are as follows.

1. The *Tu Mo,* or Channel of Control, runs along the spinal column, from the coccyx up through the neck to the skull, and over the crown of the head to the roof of the mouth.

2. The *Jen Mo,* or Channel of Function, goes through the center and front of the body. Its lower extremity is at the genital organs, and it extends up to the base of the mouth. When the tongue rests against the palate, it forms a bridge between the *Tu Mo* and the *Jen Mo.*

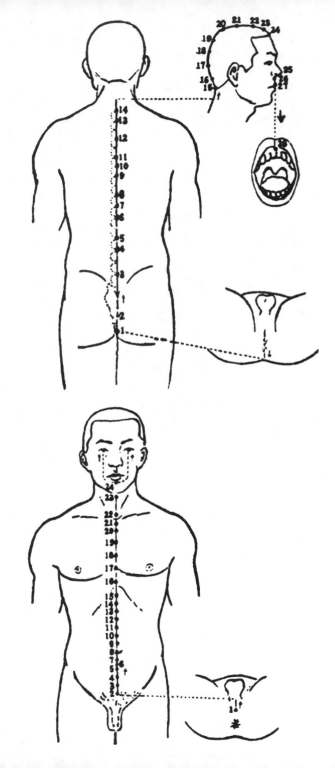

Tu Mo

Jen Mo

3. The *Tai Mo,* or Belt Channel, is so called because it circles the waist like a belt. It begins under the navel, where it divides into two branches, which extend around the waist to the small of the back.

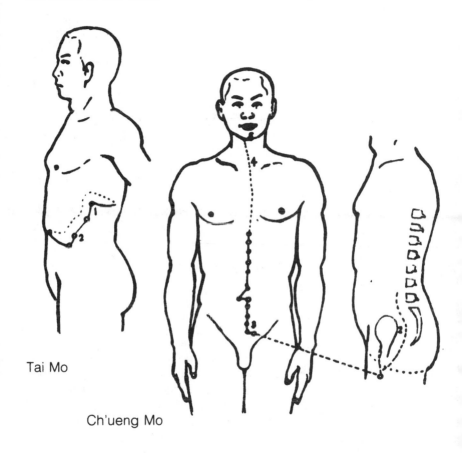

Tai Mo

Ch'ueng Mo

4. The *Ch'ueng Mo,* or Thrusting Channel, passes through the center of the body, in front of the Tu Mo and behind the Jen Mo. Its lower end is at the genitals, and it extends upward to just below the heart.

5. The *Yang Yu Wei Mo,* or Positive Arm Channel, also begins below the navel, passes through the chest to the shoulders, and goes then down the outer sides of the arms to the tips of the middle fingers, then around to the center of the palms.

6. The *Yin Yu Wei Mo,* or Negative Arm Channel, extends along in inner sides of the arms, from the palms to the shoulders, and ends in the chest.

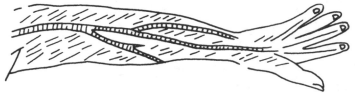

Detail from Yang Yu Wei Mo

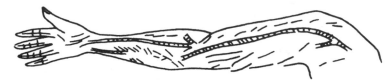

Detail from Yin Yu Wei Mo

7. The *Yang Chiao Mo,* or Positive Leg Channel, extends along both sides of the body, from the center of the soles of the feet, along the outer sides of the ankles and legs, and then farther up to the head, and ends below the ears. The lower extremities of this channel in the soles are called the *yung-ch'uan* cavities. The term *yung-ch'uan* literally means "bubbling spring."

8. The *Yin Chiao Mo,* or Negative Leg Channel, also begins in the Yung Ch'uan cavities but extends up through the inside of legs to the genitals, and then farther up the center of the body to a point between the eyebrows.

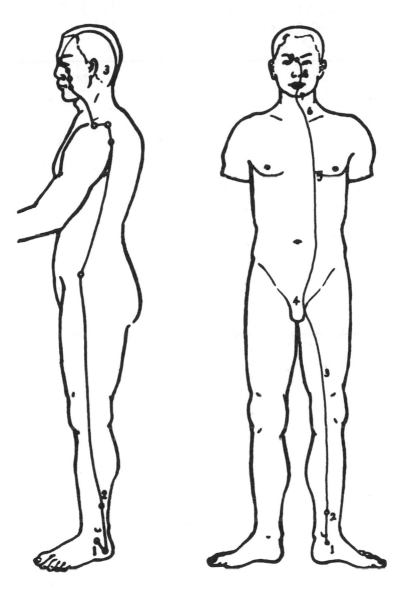

Yang Chiao Mo   Yin Chiao Mo

The eight channels together form an interconnected network of pathways through which the *ch'i* can flow freely during meditation. (Techniques for promoting this flow of energy are described in detail in later chapters.)

Perhaps the most important of the psychic channels are the Tu Mo and the Jen Mo, because along them are located the twelve psychic centers, which have special significance in meditation. Along the Tu Mo are the following centers:

wei-lu	tip of the spine
shun-fu	slightly below the middle of the spine
hsuan-hsu	middle of the spine
chai-chi	slightly above the middle of the spine
t'ao-tao	below the neck
yu-chen	back of the head
ni-wan	top of the head
ming-t'ang	between the eyebrows

Along the Jen Mo are these centers:

t'an-chung	in the chest
chung-huan	above the navel
shen-chueh	in the navel
ch'i-hai	about three inches below the navel

These psychic centers play a particularly important role in the purification of the vital energy. (Further details are given in Chapter 7, "Sitting Meditation.") The centers are symbolized in various ways in Taoist writings. They are represented by twelve hexagrams of the *I ching,* which also represent the twelve months of the year as well as the twelve times of the day. Thus the circulation of the *ch'i* through the twelve psychic centers reflects the cyclic pattern of the cosmic processes which bring about the alternation of light and darkness as well as the changing of the seasons. Harmonizing the flow of energy within the body with the cosmic processes is essential to achieving unity with the Tao, the ultimate goal of meditation.

The following diagram relates the twelve psychic centers to the twelve hexagrams that symbolize them, and indicates how the cycle reflects the times of the day and year.

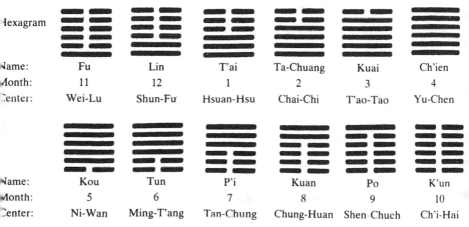

Hexagram						
Name:	Fu	Lin	T'ai	Ta-Chuang	Kuai	Ch'ien
Month:	11	12	1	2	3	4
Center:	Wei-Lu	Shun-Fu	Hsuan-Hsu	Chai-Chi	T'ao-Tao	Yu-Chen

Name:	Kou	Tun	P'i	Kuan	Po	K'un
Month:	5	6	7	8	9	10
Center:	Ni-Wan	Ming-T'ang	Tan-Chung	Chung-Huan	Shen-Chuch	Ch'i-Hai

Waxing and Waning of Ch'ien and K'un

According to Chinese astrologers the *yang* movement begins with the eleventh month, which is identified with *fu*. This *yang* movement increases through the twelfth month, *lin*, up to the fourth month, *ch'ien*, when it reaches its complete dominance. At the fifth month, *kou*, the *yang* movement begins to decrease, until, when it reaches the tenth month, *yin* has gained complete dominance. On the other hand, the *yin* movement begins to decrease in the eleventh month and this decreasing movement continues until the fourth month, when *yang* has gained complete sway. At the fifth month, *kou*, *yin* begins to increase until at the tenth month, *k'un*, it is in turn complete.

THE TWELVE MERIDIANS

In addition to the psychic channels within the body, there are twelve pathways of energy at the surface of the body, called meridians. These are connected to the internal organs by intermediate circulatory paths. The twelve take their names from the specific inner organs to which they correspond. Acupuncture and acupressure are essentially ways of regulating and balancing the distribution of energy throughout the inner organs by the manipulation of key points which lie along the twelve meridians. There are approximately a thousand of these points in all. They are of three main types: *tonification points,* through which energy can be increased in case there is a deficiency; *sedation points,* through which energy can be decreased where there is an excess, and *source points.*

Each of the meridians has a fixed direction, termed either centrifugal or centripetal. In addition, each is associated with one of the five elements, and is designated as either yin or yang, depending on the character of the energy that flows along it. The relationship between yin and yang forms of energy was described in some generality in the Introduction. Further details on regulating the balance between the two within the body are beyond the scope of this book and would require a full treatise on acupuncture. Here I will simply list the twelve meridians and describe their locations, with the aid of the accompanying diagrams. Meditation is related to human anatomy.

1. The *Lung Meridian* is yin, centrifugal in direction, and associated with the element metal. It runs along the side of the body, starting from between the second and third ribs near the armpit. From this point it goes up to the shoulder and then runs down the arm, ending at the base of the thumbnail.

2. The *Kidney Meridian* is yin, centripetal in direction, and associated with the element water. It begins on the sole of the foot, goes up the inside of the leg to the center of the body just above the genitals, and runs along the chest, ending between the collarbone and the first rib.

3. The *Large Intestine Meridian* is yang, centripetal in direction, and associated with metal. It begins at the base of the nail of the index finger, goes along the arm up to the shoulder and neck, and ends just beside the nostril.

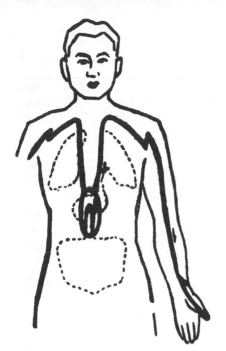

Lung Meridian

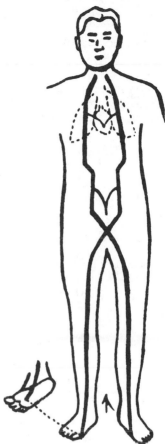

Kidney Meridian

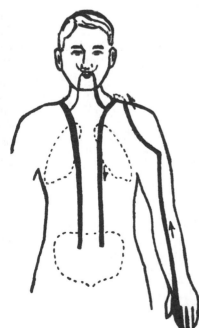

Large Intestine Meridian

4. The *Spleen Meridian* is yin, centripetal, and associated with earth. It begins at the root of the nail of the big toe, goes up along the inside of the leg and the side of the torso, and ends below the armpit.

5. The *Gallbladder Meridian* is yang, centrifugal, and associated with wood. It begins at the outside corner of the eye, passes through several points on the head, goes down the side of the body and leg, and ends at the second joint of the fourth toe.

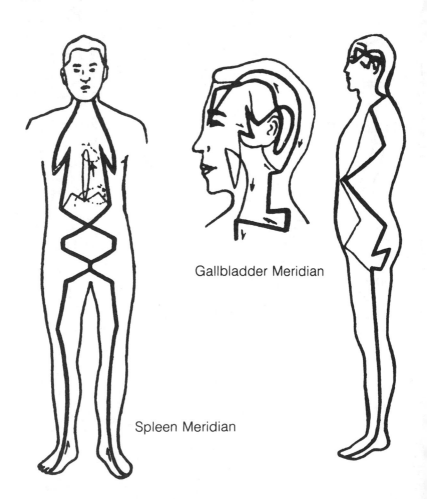

Gallbladder Meridian

Spleen Meridian

6. The *Triple Warmer Meridian* is yang, centrifugal, and associated with fire. It begins on the outer side of the ring finger (toward the little finger) and goes up the hand and arm to the head, ending just below the eyebrow.

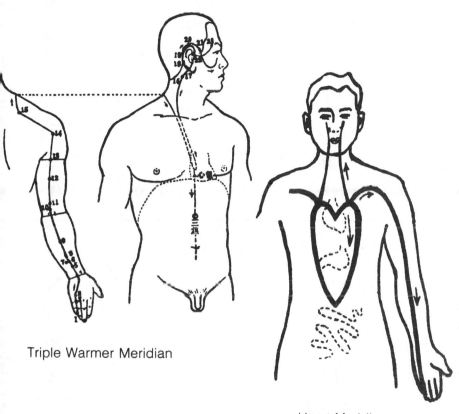

Triple Warmer Meridian

Heart Meridian

7. The *Heart Meridian* is yin, centrifugal, and associated with fire. It begins inside the armpit and goes down the inner side of the arm to the base of the little finger.

8. The *Bladder Meridian* is yang, centrifugal, and associated with water. It begins on the inside corner of the eye, goes up over the top of the skull, down the back near the spine, and down the back of the leg, ending at the base of the nail on the little toe.

9. The *Stomach Meridian* is yin, centrifugal, and associated with earth. It begins under the eye and moves down the chest and abdomen, and along the front of the leg to the base of the second toenail.

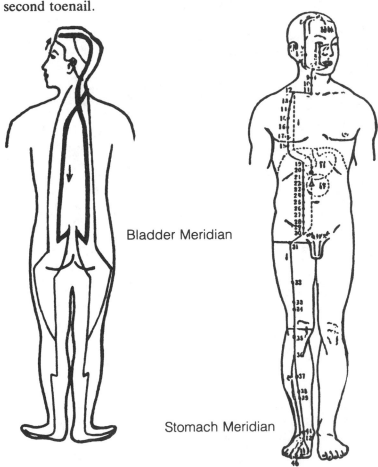

Bladder Meridian

Stomach Meridian

10. The *Small Intestine Meridian* is yang, centripetal, and associated with fire. It begins at the base of the little fingernail, goes up the arm to the side of the neck, then around to the front of the face and back over to the front of the ear, where it ends.

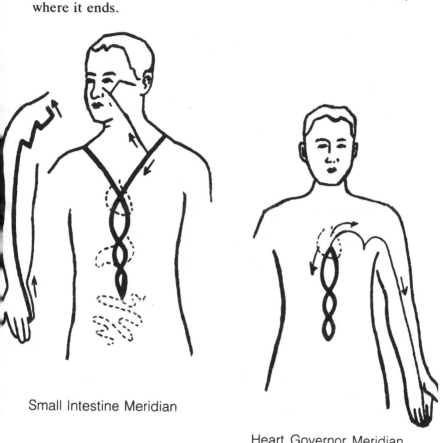

Small Intestine Meridian

Heart Governor Meridian

11. The *Heart Governor Meridian* is yin, centrifugal, and associated with fire. It begins on the chest and goes down the arm and hand to the base of the middle fingernail.

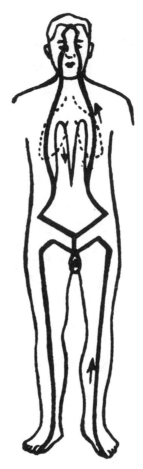

Liver Meridian

12. The *Liver Meridian* is yin, centripetal, and associated with wood. It begins at the base of the large toenail and goes up the leg and abdomen up to the chest near the nipple.

NOTE

1. Lu K'uan Yu, *Secrets of Chinese Meditation*, contains translations of some passages from Yin's treatises. See especially page 194.

CHAPTER FOUR

THE TAO OF BREATHING *(CH'I)*

Breathing has been an important subject of study in China for over five thousand years. The Taoists especially have used breathing techniques to prevent sickness, prolong youth, achieve longevity, and reach their highest goal—immortality. Many schools of martial arts, not only T'ai Chi Ch'uan, use breathing to enhance both offensive and defensive techniques. But many masters guard their secrets, never commit them to writing, passing them on orally only to sincere disciples. Perhaps this is because the subject of breathing includes many aspects that are not easily written about.

In recent years Western interest in this subject has grown, and many medical doctors are aware that deep breathing can preserve health and cure disease; but they do not describe the technique used or give detailed instructions. However, as the influence of Eastern culture has spread, many books and periodicals have mentioned this subject. Even so, until now there has been no clear and systematic description or scientific analysis of breathing techniques. In this chapter I will describe in detail the use of breathing as the foundation of meditation, T'ai Chi Ch'uan, and the Shao Lin school of martial arts.

Besides oxygen, the air that we breathe contains many elements, including iron, copper, zinc, fluorite, quartz, zincite, and magnesium. These elements supply important needs of the body. By using a combination of exercise and breathing, Taoist techniques provide an efficient and effective method for taking in these precious elements and getting rid of wastes and poisons. These techniques, as Chuang Tzu says, "expel the old, take in the new."[1] The Buddhists compare the body to a "dirty leather bag" because it contains all kinds of things—poisons, wastes, bone, tissue, and blood. The breath, properly used, can purify, repair, and clean this dirty bag. Taoist breathing techniques include not only mouth and nose breathing, but also fetal or internal breathing, discussed later in the chapter.

The Chinese word *ch'i* is always found in any description of Taoist exercise or breathing techniques. The word is represented by two ideograms, which are closely related and have the same pronunciation. The first ideogram, 氣 , gives the meaning of breathing, air, steam, or gas, and is used when we wish to indicate the atmosphere we breathe or the act of breathing—that is, taking air into the lungs, or what is called postnatal breathing in Taoist terminology. The second ideogram, 炁 , is described as being "used in Taoist charms." It refers to vital energy by transforming *ching* (liquid) to *ch'i* (steam).

The concepts of *prenatal* and *postnatal* breathing occur in Taoist writings and also are represented in diagrams such as the last one in Chapter 2. The underlying idea is as follows. Before birth, the embryo does not need to inhale and exhale, for the breath is circulated through its body from the mother. The oxygen-rich blood comes to it through the umbilical cord and enters its abdomen at the navel. Thus prenatal breathing is done through the abdomen. After birth, of course, this method of breathing is no longer available since the umbilical cord is severed. Thereafter, a person must rely on breathing through the lungs, which is thus called postnatal breathing. Most people only breathe with the throat and lungs, so that the prenatal breath hides in the abdomen, never joining the postnatal breath again. This capability plays a role in the practice of meditation, however, and so meditation and T'ai Chi Ch'uan may be said to bring about a union of prenatal and postnatal breathing. That is, during inhalation, as the meditator is drawing the postnatal breath into the lungs and down to the navel, the prenatal breath rises up from the lower abdomen to the navel, where it joins together with the postnatal breath. During exhalation, as the postnatal breath rises up out of the lungs, the prenatal breath sinks down again to the lower abdominal region. The union of prenatal and postnatal breath during meditation is figuratively represented by various images. It is referred to as the union of Fire and Water (or the union of Li and K'an). It is also described by the phrase "The sun dwells in the moon's palace." In the T'ai Chi T'u diagram reproduced at the end of the second chapter, the thin dark line in the white part of the circle represents prenatal breath, while the thin white line in the dark part of the circle represents postnatal breath. In the trigrams Li ☲ and K'an ☵, the prenatal breath is represented by the yang line between the two yin lines of K'an, and the postnatal breath by the yin line between the two yang lines of Li.

In the very advanced stages of meditation, there is a phenomenon called fetal breathing in which the meditator, like the embryo, is able to breathe without inhaling and exhaling. In this stage, which is also characterized by an absence of pulse, the meditator completely transcends conscious thought and attains a state called Great Quiescence. This is the highest form of enlightenment and the final goal of Taoist meditation. (There is a similar concept in the Buddhist meditation tradition, but different terminology is used.)

The earliest ideas about breathing are credited to Huang Ti, the Yellow Emperor. A pioneer of Chinese medical science, Huang Ti emphasized the medical and health goals of breathing. He called the technique Tu Na. *Tu* means "exhale" and *na* means "inhale." He is said to have governed for one hundred years by using these techniques. Perhaps he also used sexual methods, for Huang Ti is also reputed to have had one hundred wives. One of his female officials (or perhaps she was a concubine), Yu Nu (Jade Girl), is credited with the *Yu Nu ching,* a record of sexual techniques written in the form of questions by Huang Ti and answers by the Jade Girl. It has been translated into Japanese and English.[2] These sexual techniques, however, depend on proper breathing to achieve their goals.

The Chinese Record of History records the existence of P'eng Tzu who lived for more than eight hundred years, from the time of the Yao dynasty (2357–2283 B.C.) until sometime in the Shang Yin dynasty (1783–1054 B.C.). He is also mentioned by both Confucius and Chuang Tzu. Although little is known of his life, he is said to have developed a breathing technique which helped him achieve such a long life span.

While Lao Tzu did not specify any exercise technique, he transcribed the sounds of *fu* and *shi,* which became the basis of a system of therapeutic breathing sounds amplified by Chuang Tzu: "FU, SHU, HU and SHI—blowing and breathing with open mouth; inhaling and exhaling the breath—expelling the old breath and taking in the new. . . ."[3] Chuang Tzu contributed further definition and refinement to the development of Tao Yin: "make the climbing motions of a bear, stretch like the birds."[4] Tao Yin is not only a movement but should be combined with breathing.

A commentary on this passage from Chuang Tzu describes the nature of the movement: "Tao means guided breathing evoking harmony and Yin means the pliant and even movements of extension and contraction which make the body soft."[5] Thus rhythmical, flowing practice of the form became a vital aspect of the T'ai Chi Ch'uan.

Ch'i Wu Luen likens *ch'i* to the wind, for it goes everywhere, into every cavity of the body—not only to the mouth and nostrils, but also to the ears and the inner organs. When breathing from the Tu Mo, the Channel of Control, the *ch'i* can even reach the heels.

Mencius, a Confucian philosopher, asserted that the mind is the commander of the *ch'i* and that the *ch'i* fills up the whole body. Mencius knew how to use the *ch'i,* and he lived to be eighty-four years old, eleven years longer than Confucius. His

ideas later became a most important source of information
regarding T'ai Chi Ch'uan.

Hundreds of years after Mencius, in the Han dynasty (200
B.C.–A.D. 200), many books were written describing meditation and breathing, such as Wei Po-yang's *Ts'an tung ch'i* and
many books by Chang Tao Ling, a magician and alchemist,
who wrote much relating to meditation and magical spells.

In his book *Po pu tze,* the great alchemist Ko Hung discusses clearly and scientifically the technique of breathing.
He acquired many of his concepts by observing animals, such
as the patient turtle and the peaceful crane. In the chapter
called "Discussing the Immortals" Ko says: "The immortals
used herbs and food to nourish the body. They used the
technique [breathing and exercise] to prolong life, to prevent
sickness from developing inside the body, and to keep harm
from coming to the body from outside."[6] Physical and breathing exercises make the body healthy and strong and fortify it
against the elements. For example, on a cold day, in the
street you may see one person all bundled up with coat,
scarves, and hat, while someone else is lightly clad. The difference between the two people is that one has a healthy
body and one does not. In the same way, one person may
become ill while another person sharing the same environment will not. That is because the first person's body is not
immune to disease while the other's is. A healthy body has a
strong immunological system.

In the chapter called "Extremely Logical," Ko Hung writes:
"Everyone is in the air and the air is inside of everyone. In
heaven as well as on earth all other creatures depend on the air.
The true practitioner of breathing fortifies his body inside and
protects it from outside harm. The people use it [fetal breath-
ing] every day, but do not know it."[7] The outside air is the
atmosphere of the earth. The air inside the body is oxygen and
prenatal or fetal breathing. Everyone recognizes the importance of oxygen, but very few people are aware of prenatal
breathing. When a person dies a natural death, it is because
prenatal breathing has become exhausted. The Buddhists say,

"When the oil is finished, the lamp is black." Meditative breathing technique can increase the oil so that the lamp will always be lit—that is, it will promote longevity.

TAOIST BREATHING

We have discussed the Taoist use of breathing from the theoretical viewpoint. Now let us look at some practical exercises.

INNER BREATHING

Although this technique is usually classified as a Sitting Meditation, I treat it as a form of Standing Meditation because it can be practiced anywhere and anytime. It is especially effective when practiced in the countryside or in a garden where the air is richer in oxygen. Accompanied by movement, this technique is easy for the beginner. It can be practiced while seated in a chair or in a sleeping posture. However, the meditation posture is the most effective. (See Chapter 6, "Standing Meditation.")

I perform this technique every day. While doing it I can actually feel the blood circulating through my veins and arteries, and my feet always become very warm. For a more in-depth theoretical description of this technique, see Lu K'uan Yu's *Taoist Yoga.*

NAVEL AND TAN-T'IEN BREATHING

This technique can be practiced in the sitting, standing, walking, or sleeping posture. It can be done anywhere and as often as you wish.

Inhale, using your mind to draw in oxygen and fetal breathing to the navel. Then use your mind to carry the ch'i down to the *tan-t'ien.* Hold it there for one minute or more. Then exhale. When you feel that your whole body is relaxed, inhale. Use your mind to bring the *ch'i* through the *tan-t'ien* (the lower abdomen) to the back, then up to the top of the head and down to the mouth. (As saliva accumulates in your mouth, swallow it and send it to the abdomen.) Then exhale again and continue to practice.

After practicing this exercise for a short time, your whole body will feel relaxed and warm. You will also be able to hear the sound of gurgling in your abdomen.

BREATHING FROM THE BRAIN TO THE KIDNEYS

Most people inhale through the nose to the *tan-t'ien*, down the front of the body. This technique reverses that order, so that the breath goes up to the head and down to the lower back or kidneys.

Inhale, using your mind to draw the *ch'i* up to the forehead to the top of the head, then down through the Tu Mo (Channel of Control). Exhale to the kidneys. Then inhale again, using your mind to draw the *ch'i* up to the head and down to the nose. Then exhale. When you inhale, your mind will feel clear and calm. The kidneys are more important than either the heart or the abdomen. The Buddhists say, "The kidney is the lotus root. The heart is the lotus flower." I would add to this that the lungs are the leaves. It is more important to fertilize the root than to water the leaves and the flowers. (See illustration on page 56.)

CH'I IN THE MARTIAL ARTS

To many Westerners, the most fascinating aspect of the Eastern martial arts is the way in which they rely on the power of the *ch'i*. When the body is full of *ch'i*, it becomes very strong—as strong as the tires of a truck when they are filled with air. When the tires are full, the truck can transport heavy loads over long distances. But if the tires lose their air, they cannot even hold themselves up, much less carry the body of the truck.

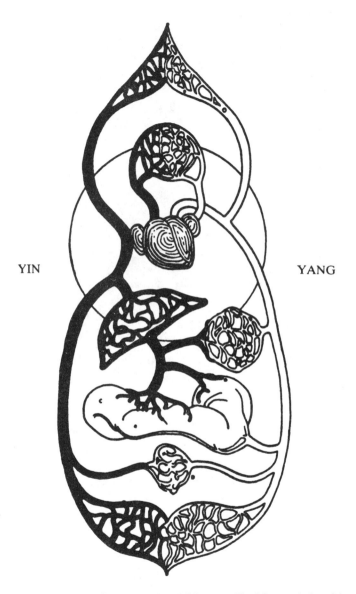

YIN   YANG

Breathing from the Brain to the Kidneys: Tu Mo and Jen Mo

SOURCE: Reprinted from *Fundamentals of Yoga* by Rammurti Mishra, M.D. Copyright © 1959 by Rammurti F. Mishra, M.A., M.D. Used by permission of The Julian Press, Inc.

The power of the *ch'i* can best be illustrated in the feats of the most advanced practitioners of the martial arts. There is a story about Moslem Sa, a Master of the Iron Clothes (so called because he was as fearless as if iron clothes protected his body), who used a large log to demonstrate his technique. The log, suspended by beams and manipulated by two strong men, would be thrust against his stomach. He remained unharmed and immobile.

The great Tai Chi Ch'uan masters also used the power of *ch'i*. Wang Tsung-yueh, in his commentary on "The Thirteen Postures," wrote: "When preparing to attack, store [inhale] the *ch'i* like drawing a bow. At the same time make the humming sound 'Hun'. When attacking, release [exhale] the *ch'i* like shooting the arrow, at the same time, make the laughing sound 'Ha.' "[8]

The story is told that once when Master Yang Chien Hou (1842–1917) was in the courtyard letting his student punch him in the abdomen, he suddenly let out the laughing sound, *Ha.* His student fell back twenty steps, so strong was the power of the *ch'i* released through this sound.

The *ch'i* must be accumulated gradually and slowly. As Chuang Tzu says of the wind, "So it is with the accumulation of wind, if it be not great, it will not have the strength to support great wings."[9] From a small breeze, the wind must gradually become a tornado. The small breeze cannot move the weak grass. But when the breeze increases to become a tornado, it can uproot trees, hurl houses into space, and knock down tall buildings. Mencius states of the *ch'i:* "It is exceedingly great and exceedingly strong. Being nourished by rectitude, and sustaining no injury, it fills up all between heaven and earth."[10]

To accumulate *ch'i* in the body, constant regular and unhurried practice of the form is required. Mencius wrote: "Let not the mind forget its work, but let there be no assisting the growth of that nature."[11] Such practice should never try to force results. Mencius continues: "Let us not be like a man of Sung [State]. There was a man of Sung, who was grieved that

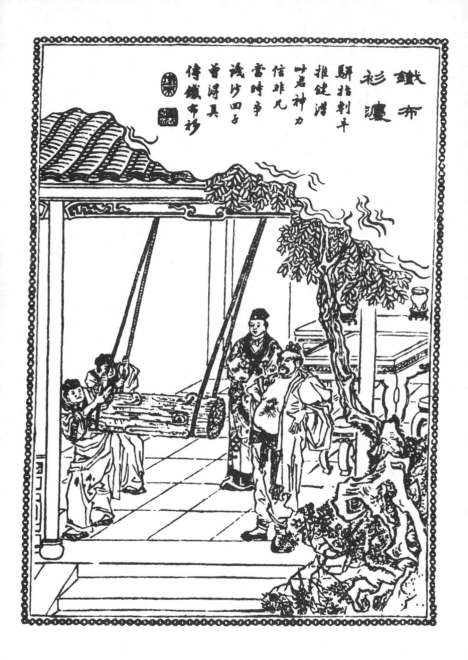

Moslem Sa demonstrates the power of *ch'i*.

SOURCE: *Liao Tza* by P'u Sun Ling, early Ching dynasty book of short stories.

his growing corn was not longer, and so he pulled it up. Having done this, he returned home, looking very stupid and said to his people, 'I'm tired today. I have been helping the corn to grow long.' His son ran to look at it, and found the corn all withered."[12]

NOTES

1. Chuang Tzu.
2. See Akira Ishihara and Howard S. Levy, trans., *The Tao of Sex* (New York: Harper & Row, 1968).
3. Chuang Tzu.
4. Ibid.
5. Lee.
6. Ko Hung.
7. Ibid.
8. Wang Tsung-yueh.
9. Chuang Tzu.
10. Mencius, *The Chinese Classics,* Vol. II, *The Works of Mencius,* trans. James Legge (Hong Kong: Hong Kong Univ. Press, 1960), p. 190.
11. Ibid.
12. Ibid.

CHAPTER FIVE

THE WAXING AND WANING OF CH'IEN AND K'UN

One of my T'ai Chi and meditation masters once remarked to me, "If you want to learn meditation, first you must read the *I ching,* the *Tao te ching,* and other works that speak of Tao." He also said that one should read books related to medicine, physiology, and human anatomy, especially those that deal with acupuncture. This knowledge is essential for an understanding of the psychic channels and spiritual centers in the body which are employed in meditation. Here we will consider the significance of the *I ching* for T'ai Chi Ch'uan and meditation.

Chinese concepts of meditation come primarily from *I ching.* These concepts are contained both in the *Great Treatise* and in the *I ching* hexagrams, the six-line figures consisting of broken and unbroken lines. In particular, the twelve "calendar" hexagrams, standing for the months of the year, are very important, since they correspond to the twelve psychic centers. They also symbolize the process of waxing and waning of Ch'ien (yang), the creative principle, and K'un (yin), the receptive principle. The *Great Treatise* states, "Therefore, they called the closing of the gates the Receptive [exhale], and the opening of the gates the Creative [inhale]. The alternation between closing and opening they called change. The going backward and forward without ceasing they called penetration."[1] According to Wilhelm, the translator of the *I ching,* the closing and opening of the gates represents the respiration.

Forward-and-backward movement is a key principle of T'ai Chi Ch'uan practice. Penetration refers to that level in meditation at which the meditator has attained mastery in the psychic as well as the physical sphere and is able to move forward and backward in time.

In the hexagrams, the increase of yang (positive) power, shown by the progression of unbroken lines from the bottom to the top of the hexagram, represents the waxing of Ch'ien and the waning of K'un. This process takes place in the first six months of the year as each succeeding hexagram adds another solid line. At the height of the yang phase, the hexagram consists entirely of solid lines, and then the yin forces (represented by broken lines) begin to increase and yang decreases. Now K'un is waxing and Ch'ien is on the wane. This process conforms to the progression of natural forces, as the whole year in its germination, growth, blossoming, fruition, and harvest is symbolically represented. The correspondence between the seasons and the process of meditation is further attested to by the title of a work on Taoist meditation, translated as *The Secret of the Golden Flower,* wherein meditation is compared to a plant that grows, falls, and is born anew.

In meditation, then, the elixir (*tan*), or spiritual force, is conceived of as a natural growth that must be cultivated. The meditation cycle begins at the center of the body known as the *tan-t'ien,* the field (*t'ien*) in which the elixir is planted. This area is located one and one-half inches below the navel. Both T'ai Chi Ch'uan and meditation employ the mind so that the breath sinks down to the *tan t'ien.* The *ch'i* (breath) is used like an ox to plow the field. Buddhist writings often refer to the *ch'i* as a big white ox that plows the field and plants the seeds, which start to germinate underground as the roots grow downward. The roots are symbolized by the first calendar hexagram, Fu, which also corresponds to the psychic center called *wei-lu,* the tip of the spine. *Wei-lu* means "the Gate of the Tail," which is where the circulation of the elixir in meditation begins.

FU

The hexagram Fu has K'un (Earth) as the upper trigram and Chen (Wood) as the lower. The two nuclear trigrams are both K'un. Thus the meaning of the whole hexagram is "roots deep under the earth." In T'ai Chi Ch'uan this hexagram represents the feet on which the T'ai Chi player stands firmly like a tree rooted in the ground. In the *Classics of T'ai Chi Ch'uan* it is said: "The energy is rooted in the feet, develops in the legs, is directed by the waist." The lower trigram (Chen) means "ascending." Thus, the vitality is guided up through the roots, the *wei-lu,* to the other psychic centers.

The hexagram Fu corresponds to the Chinese eleventh month, the time of the winter solstice when the trees are bare of leaves but their roots are beginning to stir. It is also midnight, when all is quiet and recovery is beginning. The yin, or negative, is at its lowest ebb. The yang, or positive, is beginning to rise. The Taoist believes that this is the best time to begin meditation for it is now that the inner elixir is beginning to sprout and the *ch'i* is at its most powerful.

LIN

The next calendar hexagram is Lin, which adds another unbroken line to the one solid line contained in Fu. Thus, the hexagram consists of two solid lines under four unbroken lines, representing the continued growth of yang. Here the upper trigram is K'un, while the lower trigram is Tui (Joyous). The lower nuclear trigram consisting of two broken lines above a solid line is Chen, while the upper nuclear trigram is K'un. Thus, the firm element, the solid line, is ascending and penetrating.

The Commentary on the Decision of the hexagram Lin states, "The firm penetrates and grows." In T'ai Chi Ch'uan, energy penetrates from the foot to the leg. The Commentary also says, "The firm is in the middle. . . ." Therefore, it is required that the energy be placed in the middle of the leg. Finally, the Commentary notes, " 'Great success through correctness': this is the course of heaven." In both Tai Chi Ch'uan and meditation, if the practitioner maintains a correct posture, the *ch'i* begins to rise through the channel of the spine to the front, until it reaches the *tan t'ien,* in the course known as the Greater Heavenly Circulation. The hexagram Lin corresponds to *shun-fu,* the next psychic center, after *wei-lu,* on this course.

T'AI

The next hexagram, T'ai (Peace), adds another unbroken line to its predecessor. The new hexagram consists of three unbroken lines below and three broken lines above. The lower trigram is Ch'ien (Heaven), while the upper trigram is again K'un. The hexagram T'ai is associated with the first month of the Chinese year (corresponding to February–March), which is regarded as the beginning of spring. The hexagram also stands for the next psychic center, in the lower middle of the spinal cord, the *hsuan-hsu.*

The Commentary observes, "In this way heaven and earth unite, and all beings come into union." One achieves unity through both meditation and T'ai Chi Ch'uan. The Commentary also states, "Upper and lower unite, and they are of one will." In both meditation and T'ai Chi Ch'uan, the practitioner must be of one will; he or she must concentrate without a wandering mind. The Commentary adds that "strength is within and devotion without. . . ." Thus, in practicing T'ai Chi Ch'uan, the player must be soft outside and firm inside. Finally, the three broken lines of the upper trigram indicate that the breath may pass unobstructed down to the abdomen, while the three unbroken lines of the lower trigram indicate the solidity of the lower part of the body.

One other noteworthy feature of this hexagram is the following: if we interchange the second line with the fifth line, we obtain the trigram Li (Fire) below since we have two unbroken lines containing a broken line; and we have the trigram K'an (Water) above, consisting of two broken lines containing an unbroken line. The resultant hexagram represents the union of K'an and Li. In the body, this signifies that fire, which originates in the region of the heart, goes to the place of water, in the abdomen. Thus, the *ching,* or sexual energy, is purified by fire and becomes *ch'i,* the vitality that circulates throughout the body in meditation. (Also, the heat produced in the body during T'ai Chi Ch'uan and meditation serves to evaporate excess water, which can cause many illnesses.)

TA CHUANG

The hexagram after T'ai is Ta Chuang, or the Power of the Great, which corresponds to both the second month and the next psychic center in the upper middle of the spine, known as the *chai-chi.* The upper trigram is Chen (Arousing); the lower trigram is Ch'ien, creative, strong, and firm; and the nuclear trigrams are Ch'ien and Tui (Joyous). Thus, the structure of the hexagram is very strong, analogous to the spinal cord of both the meditator and the T'ai Chi player. The unbroken lines, representing both yang and Ch'ien, are still on the increase. The *ch'i* continues its upward progress along the spinal cord.

The Commentary on this hexagram states, "Power in the toes. Continuing brings misfortune." This refers to the necessity for the T'ai Chi player to maintain balance but not to freeze in any given position. Rather, the player must make his or her movements smooth and flowing but controlled. The second line of the Commentary states, "The nine in the second place finds good fortune through perseverance because it is in a central place." This accords with the principles of both T'ai

Chi Ch'uan and meditation, namely, that one must center one's mind and body.

The third line of the Commentary reads, "The inferior man works through power. The superior man does not act thus." It also notes, "A goat butts against a hedge and gets its horns entangled." Thus, the T'ai Chi practitioner never uses muscle strength in movements or in self-defense. Rather, he or she is pliable and yielding, but strong within. The meditator, too, must not use strength of will or conscious striving to clear the mind. This will only result in further harmful ego involvement.

The fourth line of Commentary says, "The hedge opens; there is no entanglement." The T'ai Chi player who yields and gives way under attack will save himself from entanglement and harm. Finally, the Commentary notes of the goat that butts its head against the hedge, "It cannot go backward, it cannot go forward." Thus, both the T'ai Chi practitioner and the meditator are warned against losing their balance through excessive striving. The T'ai Chi player who loses balance will become entangled; the meditator who strives too hard may encounter physical and mental troubles.

KUAI

The hexagram Kuai consists of five yang lines topped by one yin. The upper trigram is Tui and the lower trigram is Ch'ien, while the nuclear trigrams are both Ch'ien. Thus, this hexagram has even greater strength than the preceding one. Since here the yang lines are about to drive out the yin, this hexagram is called Resoluteness.

The *Classics of T'ai Chi Ch'uan* state that through long and resolute practice, energy (*ch'i*) can be accumulated. Through long meditation and practice of T'ai Chi Ch'uan, the body becomes strong, while the mind becomes resolute and can act with joy.

The Commentary states, "Strong and joyous—this means

resolute and harmonious." When T'ai Chi Ch'uan is practiced consistently, body and mind achieve harmony.

The hexagram Kuai corresponds to the third month of the Chinese year, as well as the psychic center known as *t'ao-tao*, which is located at the place where the neck is joined to the body.

CH'IEN

Finally, the sixth hexagram in the series that represents the growth of yang is Ch'ien, the Creative, corresponding to the fourth month and the *yu-chen*, the psychic center located in the middle of the skull where the brain stem joins the spinal cord.

Consisting of six unbroken lines, Ch'ien represents pure positivity. The *I ching* says, "These unbroken lines stand for primal power, which is light-giving, active, strong, and of the spirit." This stage corresponds to the level of development wherein the T'ai Chi master or the meditator possesses a mind filled with spirit, a body filled with energy, and bones filled with marrow. At this stage, the practitioner is pliant but resilient as steel. A Taoist immortal of the T'ang dynasty was named Lui Ch'un Yang, or "Pure Positive." Later, in the Sung dynasty, Chang San-feng, the originator of T'ai Chi Ch'uan, was also named Ch'un Yang-tzu, "Master of the Pure Positive."

The T'ai Chi classics hold that body and mind are ultimately guided by spirit. One who overemphasizes energy will stagnate. Thus, at the highest level, the T'ai Chi master who has reached the stage of pure positivity is guided by spirit, and his body and mind become pure and resilient. The Taoists had another term for this level, calling it *chen jen,* the "true man." The Buddhists called this stage the level of *chin kong,* or "being like gold and diamonds," indestructible. (Similarly, the Sanskrit term *vajra,* meaning "diamond," is often applied to spiritual masters and also refers to the four guardians of the

Buddhist temples, giants of strength.) One at this level is un-conquerable and becomes an "immortal."

 KOU

The hexagram Ch'ien, is related to the spiritual, since the yang is continuing to ascend along the Greater Heavenly Circulation to the center called *ni-wan,* at the crown of the head. In T'ai Chi Ch'uan, when the spinal cord is erect and centered from the *wei-lu* to the *ni-wan,* the passage of the spiritual is facilitated. However, when this high point is reached, then there is a change. The yin now begins to increase and the yang decreases. This change is symbolized by the hexagram Kou (Coming to Meet), which has one broken line in the first (bottom) place.

The *ni-wan* is both the last stage of the Tu Mo, or "controlled course" of the Greater Heavenly Circulation and the beginning of the Jen Mo, or "involuntary course," down the front of the body. Thus, it is a meeting place of inhalation and exhalation and, as such, is the station where a key transformation of the *ch'i* takes place. As I have noted, at the *ni-wan* the *ch'i* is at its most positive and spiritual; it has been converted to *shen* (spirit). Now as it starts its downward path, via the involuntary course of exhalation, it begins to be converted into *shu* (emptiness). Kou, which symbolizes the onset of this transformation, has as its lower trigram Sun (Wind), which is empty.

The Commentary for Kou states that "The weak advances to meet the firm." Thus, the controlled course meets the involuntary course, inhalation meets exhalation, and *shen* begins to become *shu.* In Taoist terminology, the fire begins to retreat. In both T'ai Chi Ch'uan and meditation, the neck must be kept erect and relaxed (both weak and firm) in order for the *ch'i* to reach the top of the head and then begin its descent. (It is interesting to note, in this connection, that the Taoist categories of yang and yin bear certain similarities to the Western picture of human anatomy. For in the Western schema the blood bearing oxygen circulates through the body to the top of the head and then returns to the heart. This corresponds to the circulation of yang through the body to the top of the head and then its transformation to yin on the downward course.)

TUN

The next hexagram on the downward course is Tun (Retreat), which has two broken lines in the first and second place, continuing the growth of yin. The hexagram corresponds to the *ming-t'ang,* the center between the eyes, and to the Chinese sixth month. The upper trigram is Ch'ien (Heaven), and the lower trigram is Ken (Mountain). Thus, the image is that of a mountain under heaven. This symbolizes the proper attitude of the T'ai Chi practitioner toward both the opponent and the master. Just as heaven is out of reach of the mountain, so is the T'ai Chi practitioner out of reach of the opponent. "When the common person advances against the master, he feels the distance incredibly long. When he retreats, he feels it exasperatingly short," say the *Classics of T'ai Chi Ch'uan.*

The Commentary on this hexagram states, " 'Retreat. Success': this means that success lies in retreating." The T'ai Chi practitioner does not attempt to match strength with the opponent; rather he or she retreats and remains pliant. This retreat is not to be confused with involuntary flight; it is controlled and powerful reserve. In meditation as well the practitioner must not attempt to force things. One must not use one's imperious will, for such will not bring enlightenment.

The hexagram Tun also symbolizes the T'ai Chi posture Step Back and Repulse Monkey, a retreating sequence of movements. In this form, if the feet are kept pointing forward and the legs bent, the *wei-lu,* or Gate of the Tail, is opened, allowing the *ch'i* to pass up the spine. Thus, even in retreat the T'ai Chi player is full of vital energy.

P'I

The next hexagram, P'i, has yin increasing to the third place. This hexagram corresponds to the seventh month as well as the *t'an-chung,* in the middle of the chest. The image of the hexagram is Standstill or Stagnation. This is because the upper trigram, Heaven, and the lower trigram, Earth, do not unite but stand in opposition. This hexagram is opposite to T'ai, Peace, and illustrates mistakes to avoid in T'ai Chi Ch'uan and in meditation.

The Commentary states, ". . . heaven and earth do not unite, and all beings fail to achieve union . . . The shadowy is within, the light without; weakness is within, firmness without." This, of course, is opposite to what is required for T'ai Chi Ch'uan. Also the hexagram is top-heavy, strong above and weak below. In T'ai Chi Ch'uan the player should be pliant above the navel and firm below.

If we interchange the fifth and second lines, we have Li above and K'an below. This means heart or fire above and water below, the state of affairs corresponding to the breathing of the layman, since it does not involve the union of K'an and Li. This undisciplined behavior is not useful for converting *ching* to *ch'i.*

KUAN

The hexagram Kuan means Contemplation. It corresponds to the eighth month as well as to the psychic center called *chung-huan* located midway between the solar plexus and the navel. Since the yin line in this hexagram has increased to the fourth place, the upper trigram is Sun (Wood), the upper nuclear trigram is Ken (Keeping Still), while the lower nuclear and lower trigrams are K'un (Earth). While it would seem that this hexagram, like P'i, is top-heavy, such is not the case. The upper trigram is pliable. The image is that of a soft wood like a willow bending in the breeze (the upper trigram also stands for wind).

The hexagram is very significant for both T'ai Chi Ch'uan and meditation, where contemplation and standstill are the two main principles. By the practice of concentration on a single object and rejecting all other thoughts, also called *chih* or "stopping" the mind, the meditator calms his wandering mind and smooths out his consciousness. *Chih-kuan* was an important part of the meditative practice of the T'ien T'ai school of Buddhist meditation in China.

The principle of concentration is also important in T'ai Chi Ch'uan. The Commentary on this hexagram states, "A great view is above. Devoted and gentle." "A great view is above" means "looking forward." The T'ai Chi player should concentrate the gaze straight ahead. "Devoted" refers to concentration without tension. A gentle manner enables the student to watch the opponent and to perceive the emotions and intentions his or her face discloses.

Further, the combination of the upper trigram, Sun, signifying wind, and the upper nuclear trigram, which, in addition to its other meanings, also signifies "finger," indicates that the T'ai Chi player who has reached a certain level can, if need be, penetrate the opponent's body with inner energy through his or her finger.

Finally, we should note that this hexagram is very significant in the Taoist religion. The Commentary states, "Contemplation. The ablution has been made, but not yet the offering. Full of trust they look up to him." This refers not only to contemplation but also to religious ritual since before meditating one must cleanse one's body and mind. The Commentary continues, "Those below look toward him and are transformed. He affords them a view of the divine way of heaven. . . ." That is, the meditator offers a view of heaven and immortality. It is significant in this connection that *Kuan* also means the Taoist temple.

PO

The next hexagram, in which the yin line increases to the fifth place, is Po, associated with the Chinese ninth month and with the psychic center known as *shen-chueh* located in the navel. The hexagram has Ken (Mountain) as its upper trigram, while all the other trigrams are K'un (Earth). Since all lines but the sixth are yin, the meaning of the hexagram is Splitting Apart or Decay. But the one yang line remaining indicates that the big fruits are not yet eaten. Thus, the seeds of yang are retained even as yang is on the wane.

The Commentary for this hexagram reads, " 'It does not further one to go anywhere.' " Thus, when one is top-heavy in doing T'ai Chi Ch'uan, one should not attempt to move. Similarly, if one's mind is overactive in meditating, one cannot make progress. Since the yin or yielding element is changing the strong, so should the T'ai Chi player or the meditator give way, remain calm, and undertake nothing.

This hexagram is similar to the hexagrams T'ai, P'i, and Fu in that it indicates a time of decrease or growth, when the situation is nearing emptiness or fullness.

K'UN ☷☷

The final hexagram in the calendar series is K'un. In this hexagram all lines are yin, and thus K'un represents pure yielding, pure negativity, and pure emptiness. It corresponds to the Chinese tenth month (November–December), when the decay of fall has been accomplished but germination has not yet begun. The hexagram also corresponds to the psychic center called *ch'i-hai,* or "Sea of Breath," which is three inches below the navel.

With the hexagram K'un we have reached the end of the cycle. The fields are empty; the grains have gone to storage;

the seeds are dormant, waiting to sprout again. Thus, the positive (yang) is held in abeyance. Therefore, the body and mind of the T'ai Chi player as well as the meditator should also be empty and yielding. The breath should sink unobstructed down to the *ch'i-hai*.

Lao Tzu says, "Things appear multitudinous and varied, but eventually they all return to their common root. When they revert to the common root, there is quiescence. The state of quiescence is called the fulfillment of life."[2] Thus, the meditator and the T'ai Chi player should both try to attain a state of quiescence (yin). Out of this state, the positive (yang), which is enlightenment and spiritual power, will grow.

Thus, the *I ching* hexagrams, which mirror the yearly cycle of growth and decay, also reflect the cyclical nature of meditation (through the blossoming and decay of the elixir in the Greater Heavenly Circulation) and of T'ai Chi Ch'uan (through the cyclical alternation of movement and rest: the return to the beginning in the completion of the forms of the exercise).

NOTES

1. *I Ching,* trans. Richard Wilhelm and Cary F. Baynes, vol. II, p. 318.
2. Lao Tzu, *The Works of Lao Tzu,* trans. Chang Liu (Taipei: World Book Co.), p. 25.

CHAPTER SIX

STANDING MEDITATION

The classic methods of meditation are usually practiced in a sitting position. It is possible to meditate while standing or while moving about, however, and the practice of such methods can be traced to remote antiquity in China. Similar methods were also developed in the Yoga meditation tradition of India. In this chapter I will describe a method of meditating in a standing position in which movements of the body similar to those performed at the beginning and end of the T'ai Chi Ch'uan form are used to assist and guide the circulation of the vital energy, *ch'i*, through the eight psychic channels.

To begin meditating, you should stand with knees slightly bent, weight distributed evenly on both feet, which are positioned directly below the shoulders. The arms should hang relaxed at the sides, with palms facing backward. The mind should concentrate on the psychic center known as the *tan-t'ien*, located about an inch and a half below the navel, where the *ch'i* is originally located.

From the beginning position, breathe in slowly, at the same time gradually lifting the arms upward and forward, while straightening the knees. By the time you are fully erect, your hands should be at the level of your shoulders, palms facing down, and inhalation should be completed. During this movement, the inward breath together with the concentration of the mind lifts the *ch'i* from the *tan-t'ien* upward to the solar plexus region, where the psychic center known as *li* is located. This psychic center is in the so-called Seat of Fire, near the heart, and it is symbolized by the trigram Li, whose principal meaning is Fire.

The next step is to exhale, at the same time drawing the wrists toward the shoulders, slightly straightening the fingers, and then pressing the hands down to the sides again. As this arm movement takes place, the legs should bend slightly, returning to the original position. During this movement, the outward breath together with the concentration of the mind drives the *ch'i* downward from the solar plexus to the lower abdomen, where the psychic center known as *k'an* is located. This center is in the Seat of Water, near the kidneys, and it is symbolized by the trigram *K'an,* whose principal meaning is Water.

The upward and downward movements should be repeated many times, thus circulating the *ch'i* back and forth between the solar plexus and the lower abdomen. This is the first purification cycle, known as the Lesser Heavenly Circulation, also described as the union of fire and water. Its practice refines the *ch'i* and prepares it for the next step in its purification, in which it is circulated through all eight of the psychic channels and through all twelve of the psychic centers. This is called the Greater Heavenly Circulation. The origin of the terms "Greater" and "Lesser" is to be found in the way these cycles reflect the cyclic revolutions of the heavenly bodies. The Lesser Heavenly Circulation refers to the movements of the sun and moon, which occur in the course of a single day and night. The Greater Heavenly circulation refers to the pattern of movements that occur in the course of an entire year.

The same movements described above can be used to guide the beginning of this circulation, through the proper concentration of the mind. During the inhalation and upward movement, the *ch'i* is experienced as moving first downward from the *tan-t'ien,* through the Gate of Mortality at the very bottom of the trunk, and back into the lower extremity of the Channel of Control (Tu Mo) at the coccyx, and then upward along this channel through the spinal column to the crown of the head. During the exhalation and downward movement, the *ch'i* is experienced as moving down from the top of the head to the base of the mouth, where it enters the Channel of Function

(Jen Mo), and then down through this channel, which passes through the center of the body to the Gate of Mortality.

In order to continue the Greater Heavenly Circulation, moving the *ch'i* through the remaining six psychic channels, you should proceed as follows. The next inhalation drives the *ch'i* into the Belt Channel (Tai Mo), which circles the waist like a belt. While breathing in slowly, raise the arms until the hands are at the level of the navel. This helps to lift the *ch'i* from the Gate of Mortality to the *tan-t'ien,* where it enters the Belt Channel. While continuing to inhale, move the elbow back gently as the *ch'i* divides in two branches just below the navel and moves around both sides of the belly to the small of the back. Still continuing to breathe in, lift the arms and unbend the knees to bring the *ch'i* up the back, where the Belt Channel finally ends at the scapulae.

As the breath moves out again, the movements of the arms and legs are the same as in the first exhalation. This time, however, the mind concentrates on letting the *ch'i* flow from both shoulders down the Positive Arm Channels (Yang Yu Wei Mo) along the outside of the arms, across the backs of the hands to the tips of the fingers, ending in the middle of the palms.

The next step is to lift the *ch'i* from the palms into the Negative Arm Channels (Yin Yu Wei Mo) along the inside of the arms and up to the scapulae again. This is done by breathing in, at the same time repeating the arm and leg movements of the first inhalation.

As you exhale again, once again repeating the downward movements of the arms and legs, the *ch'i* moves down from the shoulders to just below the navel, where its two branches are united again, and then down farther to the genital region. Here it is ready to enter the Thrusting Channel (Ch'ueng Mo).

The Thrusting Channel goes up from the genitals, passing through the center of the body between the Channel of Control and the Channel of Function, and ends at the solar plexus just below the heart. To lift the *ch'i* through this channel, one should inhale and repeat the upward movements of the arms and legs. It is very important, however, that the *ch'i* not be raised higher than the solar plexus. To ensure that it does not rise too high, one should be careful not to raise the hands above the level of the diaphragm during this inhalation.

The next exhalation sends the *ch'i* down again, this time to the genital region, where it divides in two and descends further into the Positive Leg Channels (Yang Chiao Mo) along the outer sides of the legs and ankles, across the tops of the feet to the toes, and then under to the Yung Ch'uan cavity located in the soles of the feet. While breathing out, one repeats the downward movements of the arms and legs.

From the Yung Ch'uan cavities, the *ch'i* rises into the Negative Leg Channels (Yin Chiao Mo) along the inner sides of the legs, through the genitals, where it unites again, and then up to the *tan-t'ien*. To accomplish this, one inhales while unbending the knees and raising the arms until the hands are at the level of the navel.

The final exhalation sends the *ch'i* down to the Gate of Mortality again, and the arms and legs resume the beginning position. This completes one cycle of the Greater Heavenly Circulation.

Regarding this process, certain points should be emphasized in order to prevent misunderstanding. First, the circulation of the *ch'i* through the psychic channels does not occur automatically as a result of the arm and leg movements and the breathing. Rather, it is the mind's power of concentration that combines with the breathing to move the *ch'i* through the channels. The outer movements aid and guide the inner concentration. Such aid can be extremely helpful, particularly to beginners, for promoting the experience of the circulation of the *ch'i*. It is not necessary, however. The Greater Heavenly Circulation can be practiced without any outer movement, purely by the power of inner concentration and breathing, in either a standing or seated position.[1]

Second, the guiding movements I have described are those of the very beginning of the T'ai Chi Ch'uan form. But as I have already mentioned, T'ai Chi Ch'uan may be accurately regarded as a method of moving meditation. Many of the other movements of the T'ai Chi Ch'uan form are just as effective as the beginning for promoting the circulation of the *ch'i* through the psychic channels. This is particularly true of movements such as White Crane Spreads Wings, Needle at the Bottom of the Sea, Play Arms Like a Fan, Fair Lady Works at Shuttle, and Wave Hands Like Clouds.[2]

NOTES

1. See Lu K'uan Yu, *Taoist Yoga,* chap. 3.
2. Details about how to use these and other movements to guide the Greater Heavenly Circulation can be found in my book *T'ai Chi Ch'uan and I Ching* (New York: Harper & Row, 1978), especially on pp. 81–83.

CHAPTER SEVEN

SITTING MEDITATION

The traditional method of meditation, which is specifically mentioned in the ancient Taoist classics, is practiced in a seated position. It involves no regular movement of the limbs, such as that of the standing techniques in the preceding chapter. The circulation of the *ch'i,* which the movement of the limbs tends to encourage, is achieved by the method of breathing and mental concentration alone. Although the sitting method is more difficult for the beginner, it is more convenient in the advanced development of the practice.

The mental concentration required for meditation is subtle. The Taoist classics suggest that it is not possible to attain it by focusing one's attention on any definite object or specific content; one should forget everything, think of nothing. Although this is a profound truth, one must take care not to misinterpret such sayings. Anyone who has tried it knows that it is very difficult to empty the consciousness of all thoughts at will. Even after becoming very placid, one is likely to find that many random ideas and distractions force their way in and that it is very hard to get rid of them without introducing other thoughts, for even the idea of abstaining from thought is itself a thought.

There has been some discussion of this problem in Western philosophical literature, and some writers have argued that it is impossible to empty the mind completely of thoughts. It is important to realize, however, that nothing like this is involved or required in Taoist meditation. The state of emptiness and total forgetfulness described in the classics refers to the final goal and highest level of the practice of meditation, the attainment of the state known as the Great Quiescence. For the beginner, it is a mistake to try to fight against distractions or drive away all thoughts. Rather, the point is to concentrate on the processes involved in meditation: the slow, rhythmic breathing and the flow of energy through the psychic channels. Focusing the attention on these things has the effect of quieting the mind and enables the meditator to forget—at least temporarily—the cares, worries, and thoughts of ordinary daily life. Thus a certain peacefulness and sense of emptiness are benefits that can be felt even in the early stages of the practice of meditation. Advanced development of this experience, however, requires daily practice over a long period of time, and it cannot be accomplished at will or be forced.

This chapter describes how to begin the practice of Sitting Meditation and discusses some traditional ways of thinking about progress and improvement in this practice.

PROPER CONDITIONS FOR MEDITATION

Not all places and times are equally suitable for the practice of meditation. For the beginner, it is especially important to practice in a quiet place. As you become more experienced, it is easier to ignore the stray noises that may create serious problems when you are just starting. The place should not be too cold, windy, or humid. Care should be taken that the room be clean and uncluttered, and that it be neither too light nor too dark. Bright, direct light should be especially avoided, for it disturbs concentration. It is an advantage if there are plants nearby, since they give off oxygen. Pets and other animals are undesirable, however, since they are sources of noise, dirt, and germs. If there are distracting smells, they can be driven away by burning incense. The surface for sitting should be cushioned so that you can sit for a long time without discomfort, but it should provide firm support. A wooden platform covered with a couple of layers of blankets is ideal. The clothing and belt should be loose enough so that one can breathe deeply with ease. Since a full stomach interferes with the flow of energy as well as with breathing, avoid eating for an hour or two before meditating. So as not to become too thirsty, however, you may partake moderately of tea or warm water.

Traditionally, the best time to practice meditating is between 11:00 P.M. and 1:00 A.M., at the beginning of the yang time of the day. Many people find, however, that because of their personal schedules and working hours, it is necessary to sleep during this period. For them, it is usually just as effective to meditate soon after rising in the morning.

HOW TO BEGIN

Having made adequate preparations, you start simply by assuming the correct seated position and beginning slow, deep breathing. The correct sitting posture is very important. The body should be erect, with spine straight and head centered. The eyes should be open, but not too widely, and focused downward on the tip of the nose. The nose should be in line with the center of the body. The mouth should be closed gently, and the tongue should lightly touch the palate. The shoulders should be relaxed and balanced at the same horizontal level. The arms should be relaxed and bent at the elbows.

The hands should be clasped together so as to form the T'ai Chi T'u symbol: (1) Touch the middle finger of the left hand with the tip of the right thumb. (2) Bring the left thumb down over the right thumb and allow it to touch the inside of the first joint of the left middle finger. (3) Curve the fingers of the left hand slightly and clasp the right hand around the left.

There are three different leg positions that may be considered correct. Experienced meditators usually sit in a full lotus position. For the beginner or aged person whose joints may not be flexible enough to assume this posture with ease, it is just as well to simply cross the legs tailor-style at first. As

Full-Lotus Posture

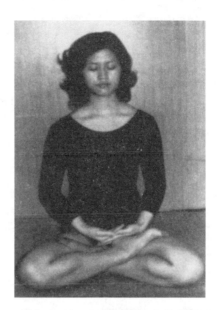

Half-Lotus Posture
Right leg over left leg.   Left leg over right leg.

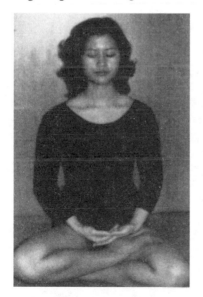 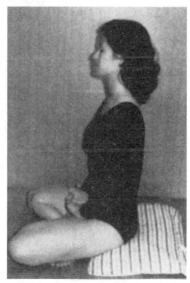

SOURCE: Chu/Nan. *Tao and Longevity*. Samuel Weiser, Inc. York Beach, ME. 1984. Used by permission.

you grow more accustomed to sitting, it will gradually become possible to get into a half-lotus position, and before long, a full lotus. It is better to be comfortable than to force the tendons and ligaments to stretch beyond their natural capacities. Such forcing can result in pain in the legs that will interfere with the concentration of the mind.

Beginners often find that sitting in the same posture for a long time interferes with the circulation of their legs, causing numbness that is painful and distracting. If one perseveres, however, after a few weeks the numbness subsides by itself. It then becomes possible to sit for hours without discomfort. In the meantime, there are always ways to alleviate the pain. One is to stretch the legs out in front of you, close together but not touching, clasp both hands together, and raise them above your head, palms outward. Another is to stand on the right leg and briskly shake both the left foot and left hand. Alternate legs. Both of these methods result in an immediate local increase of blood flow to the legs.

Even more important than correct posture is the proper method of breathing. It is essential to breathe in a way that is conducive to the flow of vital energy through the body and to the attainment of a peaceful mind. Before beginning a period of meditation, exhale vigorously through the mouth. This expels all the stale air in the lungs. According to a traditional Taoist practice, one should exhale six times, using the mouth to form a different sound each time. This is called Six Sounds for the Benefit of Inner Organs.[1] After this exhalation, one should begin regular breathing through the nose. The breathing should be slow and thin, so as to make no sound. It should be even and rhythmic. As an aid in maintaining the slow steady rhythm, it is helpful to count the breaths. One inhalation and one exhalation together count as one breath. One can count from one to ten and then repeat or, if it is easier, to fifty or to a hundred. Counting is also helpful for avoiding daydreams and other distractions. Gradually, the distinctness of the distracting thoughts will fade as the slow monotony of the counting takes over. In using such a method, be careful not to become so quiet as to be overcome by drowsiness and fall asleep. Meditation requires an alert and clear mind.

The breathing should be deep so that the air fills the abdomen, not the chest. Most people generally breathe in a very shallow manner, as if they were drawing the air no farther than the throat. When they try to breathe deeply, they usually distend the chest and become puffed out. The method of deep breathing necessary for meditation is much more relaxed. It directs air to the center of the abdomen, the *tan-t'ien*.

After becoming reasonably comfortable with the posture and the breathing, the beginner should start concentrating on the flow of vital energy in the body. At first this is a matter of using the concepts of the psychic channels as well as the Lesser and Greater Heavenly Circulation. The meditator consciously thinks of the flow of energy through the cycles that run from heart to kidneys and along the spine. Both currents are incorporated in the Greater Heavenly Circulation, which passes the *ch'i* through all the psychic centers in coordination with the rhythm of the breathing. Eventually the meditator begins to feel the breath generating a powerful warmth, which spontaneously circulates throughout the body. This indicates that the process of purification of the vital energy is taking place. Considerable practice is needed in order to develop this perception. Thus, the beginner should not be impatient for results and should not overdo his practice. Genuine progress comes after the practice has been established as a habit that fits naturally into the daily routine.

After a period of meditation, it is good to continue sitting briefly before rising and going about your activities. Exhaling through the mouth at this time helps to disperse the warmth caused by the meditation and enables the body to recover its normal temperature. You should also shake the head and move the arms about gently to normalize the blood circulation. After a few moments, you are able to begin your usual activities with renewed vigor, feeling greatly refreshed.

PROGRESS AND IMPROVEMENT
IN MEDITATION PRACTICE

Progress in this practice comes very slowly and requires faithfulness and perseverance. It is essentially a process of energy purification in which *ching* is transformed into *ch'i,* which can be circulated through the eight psychic channels when it combines with the breath. The circulation of the *ch'i* purifies it, ultimately transforming it into *shen* (spirit). At the highest level, *shen* becomes *shu* (emptiness). But in order to notice the results of the refinement process, one must circulate the *ch'i* throughout the cycle of channels many times. Thus I emphasize that it is necessary to make the practice of meditation an integral part of one's daily life. This is not only a matter of finding time to practice each day. Meditation eᵢ - genders attitudes that affect one's life-style in a variety of ways. Like everyone else, the meditator relies on food for nourishment as well as for energy. Since the meditation process is one of energy refinement, it cannot be carried on successfully if the meditator runs out of energy because of insufficient nourishment. Hunger is painful and interferes with the concentration of the mind during meditation. On the other hand, if the stomach is stuffed and there is difficulty of digestion, the flow of energy in the abdominal region is greatly hindered. Thus, the dedicated student of meditation will develop the habit of eating food that is nutritional and easy to digest, such as brown rice and vegetables. To be avoided are sweets, spicy foods, alcohol, and rich foods of any sort. It is also wise to eat in moderation. In other aspects of life as well, devotion to the practice of meditation leads to moderation, especially with respect to frivolous expenditures of energy.

After a daily practice has been well established, the meditator will gradually begin to notice improvement, which can be perceived in definite stages. At first, one cannot feel the circulation of the *ch'i* spontaneously and must rely instead on the

conscious imagination to think through the cycle in coordination with the breathing. After this practice is repeated for a
long time, however, a flow of warmth up the back and down
the front of the body can be felt independently of conscious
thought. This is the second stage of development. At a more
advanced stage, a much more powerful feeling is experienced.
The abdomen becomes very hot, and one suddenly feels a
surge of vital energy go back into the base of the spine, then
up the Tu Mo to the top of the head. As it comes over the top
of the head and enters the Jen Mo, a flow of very clean and
sweet-tasting saliva is felt in the mouth. This is distilled from
the *ch'i,* which then flows down the Jen Mo in the form of
water. This flow of saliva is often called divine nectar in Taoist
writings on meditation. Other phenomena that may be perceived at the more advanced stage include a vibration in the
belly, a shaking of the whole body, and an involuntary motion
of the limbs. These side effects are not essential to the meditation process, however. You may or may not perceive them,
depending on your age and physical constitution.

Taoist literature and art use several different images to describe metaphorically the progress of meditation and its results. The three stages of progress mentioned here are described in a particularly fanciful way in a meditation treatise
entitled *Hsin Ming Kuei Ch'i,* dating from the Ming dynasty.
There, the experience of the meditator is represented by a cart
that is pulled by different animals at different stages of its
journey. In the first stage, during which conscious thought is
required, the cart is pulled by a sheep. In the second stage,
during which a flow of warmth is perceived, it is pulled by a
reindeer. In the third stage, it is pulled by a cow. The cow,
which also has symbolic importance for the Buddhist tradition,
plays a role in other Taoist images as well. (See illustration on
page 86.)

The result of the purification of the *ch'i* is often characterized as a growing plant. Tracing its stages of growth, it begins
as a yellow sprout, develops through a stem and leaf stage,
and matures into a golden flower, which finally produces

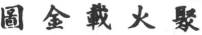

The Three Stages of Progress

SOURCE: *Hsin Ming Kuei Ch'i*, vol. I.

seeds. This analogy can be found in a book that has found some popularity in the West, *The Secret of the Golden Flower,* translated by Richard Wilhelm. It also occurs in a very interesting picture that was carved long ago in relief in stone at the Taoist temple Po Yuen Kuan (White Cloud Temple) on Beijing's West Mountain. (See illustration on page 88.) The picture outlines the seated body of a meditator. A stream of water represents the flow of energy up the Tu Mo. The *tan-t'ien,* where the *ch'i* originates, is pictured as a field of crops. In the field, a cow is pulling a plow. This represents the breath, which prepares and helps in the purification of the *ch'i* just as plowing a field prepares and helps in the growth of plants. The picture also shows water wheels at the bottom of the abdominal cavity. These are used in the irrigation of the plants and symbolize the use of concentration to send the vital energy down through the K'an region ("Seat of Water") to the base of the spine where it enters the Tu Mo.

These images are not the only ones present in the picture. Its imagery is quite complex. It also includes a number of poems to explain and further develop the significance of the images. Although I cannot fully describe these details here, let me develop the agricultural analogy a bit further and point out how it fits in with the idea that the cyclical pattern of the year is reflected in the circulation of the *ch'i.* In Taoist writings, the twelve psychic centers, mentioned in Chapter 3, are often represented by constellations of the zodiac. These zodiacal signs also stand for the twelve months of the year. Therefore, the repeated circulation of the *ch'i* through its purification cycle reflects the recurring cycle of the seasons.

Because of the cycle of the seasons, plants develop from sprout to flower to seed—themselves in a cyclic pattern that is coordinated with the seasons. If they are properly and faithfully tended, the crops will improve each year. This improvement is generally gradual, its rate depending on such factors as weather and soil conditions. But another determinant is the skill of those who care for the plants.

Similarly, if meditation is practiced faithfully each day, the

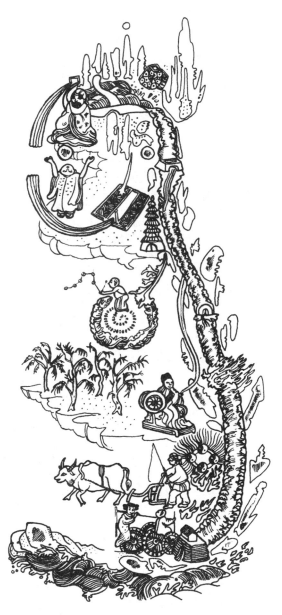

Stone Engraving in White Cloud Temple, Peking

SOURCE: Rendered by Thomas Sperling. © 1986 by Thomas Sperling. Used by permission.

result of the *ch'i* purification cycle will gradually improve. The actual rate of improvement cannot be generally predicted, however, and depends on such factors as the age and physical health of the meditator, as well as his or her wisdom.

An even more revealing analogy is used repeatedly in the classic treatises of Taoist meditation. It compares the processes by which psychic energy is refined to alchemical procedures. Alchemy was highly developed in ancient China. There were many complex procedures, but the practice mainly involved combining elements and then purifying the mixture by heating it repeatedly in various vessels. The analogy compares the body of the meditator to a laboratory in which such a purification process is taking place. The twelve psychic centers located along the psychic channels are like flasks in which the energy is refined. The breath is like wind and fire, as a bellows generates and regulates the intensity of heat applied to the flasks. The psychic energy is like the fluid mixture that is gradually purified by the successive heatings of each flask.

The stages of meditation are like those of the alchemical process. First the elements are mixed together. The body combines the nutritious substances taken from food together with various fluids secreted by the glands and inner organs. This forms both blood and the sexual essence (*ching*). Next the heat is applied to the mixture: the warmth of the breath transforms the sexual energy into *ch'i*. Then the mixture goes through a purification cycle by being passed from one heating flask to another. The *ch'i,* in other words, circulates through all twelve of the psychic centers as it moves up the Tu Mo to the crown of the head and then down the Jen Mo to return to the abdomen. The diagram on p. 93 illustrates the location of the twelve psychic centers. It shows how the *ch'i* is able to pass through them as it circulates up and down the main psychic channels.

The alchemical procedure reaches its conclusion when the refined product is taken from the flask and is either stored or used. Thus, in meditation, the product of the *ch'i* purification cycle, or *shen* (spirit), is generated eventually—after many cycles—as the *ch'i* comes up the Tu Mo to the top of the head. There, this extremely concentrated form of psychic energy can be used in various ways, or else it can continue to flow down the Jen Mo to the abdomen. By continuing its circulation, this dynamic energy can be stored up for future use.

NOTE

1. The Six Sounds—HA (beneficial to the heart), HU (spleen), SH (solar plexus), SS (lungs), SHU (liver), and FU (kidneys)—are discussed in my *Taoist Health Exercise Book* (New York: Quick Fox, 1974), p. 62.

THE FIVE CONCENTRATION POINTS

In meditation, you should concentrate mentally and physically on a specific point in order to achieve your goal. The various schools of meditation emphasize different points. Even within the same school, different masters have conflicting ideas. Actually, each point has special importance. Concentration focused on a specific point will produce a different feeling and result. I recommend that the serious meditator select one or two points and master them step by step.

1. *Ni-wan.* From the top of the head downward, the first point is the *ni-wan,* located in the crown of the head. This point is called *pei-wui* in Chinese acupuncture. *Pei* means "one hundred," and *wui* means "meeting." Many arteries, veins, and nerve endings meet at this point in the head. In Yoga it is called the *sahasrara* or crown *chakra.* When you begin to concentrate on this point, you will feel that your skin is very tight. Later on, you will feel sweat and moisture. According to Taoist belief, when you reach the highest level of meditation, your spirit leaves the body at this point. You will feel brightness on your head like the sun. The Taoist patriarch Lu Tuan Pin said that if you concentrate on this point, you will feel that your mind is very bright inside and like an inner white glow.

Some schools of meditation locate this point a little forward at the "soft spot," or fontanel, of the newborn baby. Lao Tzu calls this point the Gates of Heaven.

2. *Tzu-chiao.* The second point is located inside the

center of the head between and a little beneath the eyebrows. It is called the *tzu-ch'iao*. By concentrating your mind and half closing your eyes, you can look inside. In Western anatomy, this point is known as the pituitary gland. In Yoga it is called the Third Eye, or *ajna chakra*. By concentrating on this point, you can produce hormones and ultimately produce the elixir. There have been several recent articles on this phenomena indicating the importance of this point. In Taoist terminology, the point is known as the upper *tan-t'ien*.

3. *Chung-kung:* The Middle *Tan-t'ien.* The third point, located between the breast bone and the solar plexus, is called *chung-kung,* which means the Central Palace, or the "middle *tan-t'ien.*" In India it is called the *anahata* or heart *chakra*. In ancient times, this point was considered to be the location of the heart. At that time the heart and mind were considered as one. However, later scholars denied that the mind was located in the heart. This point is in the same location as the thymus gland according to the Western anatomy. The thymus gland is very important in regulating the immunization system of the body. In Taoist terminology this point corresponds to the trigram Li (Fire). In meditation this point (fire) combines with the fourth point (water) to produce heat, which warms the abdomen.

4. The Lower *Tan-t'ien.* The fourth point, the lower *tan-t'ien,* is called in Yoga the *manipura* or navel *chakra*. This point is located one and one-half inches (some texts say three inches) below the navel. It is 70 percent in the middle from the front and 30 percent from the back in an area somewhere between the kidney and the navel. It corresponds to the trigram K'ai. Water and sperm or eggs are produced in this area. As suggested above, concentration on this point in meditation combines fire and water, heart and kidney. When mastery is achieved, elements from all the inner organs are combined to produce sperm or egg cells, which are transformed into an elixir or "medicine." In the second phase of this chemical process, the elixir is transformed into *ch'i,* or vitality. This process produces a cavity called *ch'i-hsueh.* Most meditators

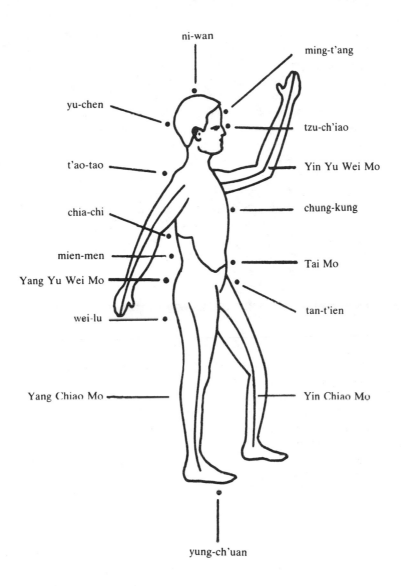

ni-wan

ming-t'ang

yu-chen

tzu-ch'iao

t'ao-tao

Yin Yu Wei Mo

chia-chi

chung-kung

mien-men

Tai Mo

Yang Yu Wei Mo

tan-t'ien

wei-lu

Yang Chiao Mo

Yin Chiao Mo

yung-ch'uan

A Diagram of Spiritual Center

use this point of concentration in the beginning. Concentration on this point gives peace of mind, warms the abdomen, and strengthens the *ch'i*. The mind then passes the *ch'i* through the fifth point to the spinal column to achieve the Greater Heavenly Circulation. This process often occurs automatically. Many Taoists refer to this area as the stove or cauldron, where fire heats water, which, when it becomes hot enough, produces vapor.

5. *Yang-kuan.* The fifth point is called *yang-kuan,* or the Cavity of Life or Death. It is similar to the Indian Muladhara or root *chakra.* It is located between the anus and the pubic region. This area is a turning point for circulating *ch'i.* When the vitality produced through meditation reaches this point, it can flow out as sperm, and when it is combined with the egg, conception takes place. Conception means birth for the baby but death for the man (or woman) because loss of vitality shortens life. If, however, the *ch'i* or vitality goes through the point and returns through the spinal column to circulate again within the body, life can be prolonged and eventually immortality will be achieved.

The meditator may use any of the points of concentration in any order. According to the book *Taoist Yoga,* the meditator should start with the second point, *tzu-ch'iao.*[1] When the goal has been achieved through concentration on this point, the meditator should combine concentration on the second point with the fourth point—the lower *tan-t'ien.* In *Secrets of Chinese Meditation* the Taoist Master Yin Shih Tzu advocated starting with the lower *tan-t'ien* (fourth point) and the shifting the concentration to the middle *tan-t'ien* (third point).[2]

NOTES

1. Lu K'uan Yu, *Taoist Yoga,* pp. 9–20.
2. Lu K'uan Yu, *Secrets of Chinese Meditation,* p. 167.

CHAPTER NINE

BREATHING MEDITATION FOR HEALTH

The purposes of meditation are to improve health and prolong life. Elements or conditions inside the body threaten health and long life more seriously than do outside agents or injuries. These inner elements are dangerous because people so often underestimate them. Those who suffer from illness of the inner organs feel only minor discomfort at first. They put off consulting a doctor until the organs have reached a critical stage of damage. By this time, it is often too late to correct the disease without costly medicines or surgery. More severe illness of the inner organs may prove fatal. The expense in terms of money, time, and suffering that results from internal disorders can be minimized or avoided through proper meditation techniques.

The source of diseases must be identified. Stagnation of the inner organs wears down the body's resistance to bacteria and viruses. These inner elements are then able to attack the inner organs more easily. Tuberculosis in the lungs, ulcers in the digestive tract, and cancer are but some of the diseases of the inner organs that can result.

We can use meditation methods to prevent such diseases. Our objectives are twofold: (1) to keep the inner organs clean and free of germs, and (2) if germs are already present, to remove them from the inner organs. The Taoist approach to cleansing the inner organs of germs is Quick Breathing. Short, quick breaths like the panting of a dog over a period of several minutes draw out the inner elements and dispose of them through the tear ducts and the mucous membranes of the nose. A similar treatment is popular in Yoga.

The form of meditation that uses Quick Breathing has changed somewhat over the centuries. In ancient times the Taoists burned sticks of incense, focused the gaze on the glow of the burning tip, and breathed very quickly until tears formed. The harmful inner elements were thus expelled through the tears. Other germs were excreted by means of mucus from the nose. However, the smoke from the incense had disadvantages, for it stimulated the eyes from the outside, not the inside, and hurt them; it also induced coughing. In place of incense, a crystal ball or hypnotist's sphere was used. The ball's smooth surface reflected light into which the meditator gazed.

I perform this meditation twice a day—when I first get up in the morning and before retiring at night. However, I do not use a crystal ball, as such equipment is difficult to find in most stores and is not necessary as such. I use a burnt-out light bulb attached to a bamboo stick or a cardboard cylinder about a foot to sixteen inches long. At this length, the ball can be held at eye level about one to two feet from the face. A tennis ball or the like will not do, since the sphere must reflect light. I concentrate my eyes on the bulb and breathe quickly through my nose for several minutes, until tears and mucus are expelled. Some of my students have complained that sustained Quick Breathing over a period of seven to ten minutes requires a great deal of energy. Six minutes is sufficient.

Quick Breathing is similar to agitating water, whereas Slow Breathing calms and restores. When Quick Breathing takes effect, the harmful inner elements are removed through the eyes and nose, the senses hum with energy, and a great amount of body heat is produced. It is now important to lower this raised body temperature and restore the body to a more natural state. I breathe slowly through the nose, directing the mind and breath and vitality back down to the abdomen. As the body resumes a calmer state, the mind experiences uncommon serenity.

The ratio between Quick Breathing and Slow Breathing is about five to one. If I perform Quick Breathing for, say, six minutes, this is followed by about half an hour of Slow Breathing. After practicing this meditation over a period of years, I have found that my eyes remain clear, I cough up less phlegm, and my body feels healthy.

Furthermore, as explained in *Taoist Yoga,* "This concentration should last until the concepts of the self and others is completely wiped out and body and mind no longer exist. Only then can your concentration be effective."[1]

NOTE

1. Lu K'uan Yu, *Taoist Yoga,* p. 44.

CHAPTER TEN

T'AI CHI CH'UAN MOVEMENTS FOR MEDITATION

In Chapter 6 I described a method of meditating in a standing posture. An important feature of the method is its use of movements of the arms and legs to assist the breathing and inner concentration that guide the *ch'i* through the psychic channels of the body in the cycles known as the Lesser and Greater Heavenly Circulations. Both the movements of the limbs and the way they are coordinated with the breathing cycle are exactly the same as those which constitute the beginning and end of the T'ai Chi Ch'uan form. The movements are rather simple, involving only the bending and unbending of the knees while the hands are lowered and raised. Yet if practiced in the way I have described, they can be very effective in directing the circulation of the *ch'i* through all of the psychic channels. What this shows is not merely that the processes of energy refinement essential to meditation can be carried out while moving as well as at rest, but, even more important, that if the external movements of the body are coordinated with inner concentration and breathing, they can assist the flow of vital energy necessary for these refinement processes to take place.

Several kinds of movement of the body and limbs in addition to those already described have also been found to be very effective for assisting the flow of the *ch'i* in meditation. Many of these are included among the several parts of the T'ai Chi Ch'uan form, which involve movements such as shifting the weight from one leg to another, rotating the body to the right or left, taking a step, moving forward or backward, and various hand and foot movements, all put together and coordinated in more or less complicated combinations and sequences.

I have studied the work of Chang San-feng, the Taoist immortal who invented T'ai Chi Ch'uan, and I believe the reason for his great achievement is that he practiced both T'ai Chi Ch'uan and meditation. The story is told that one day as he was meditating he saw a snake[1] emerge from a hole, and then a bird flew down from a tree to fight with the snake. After

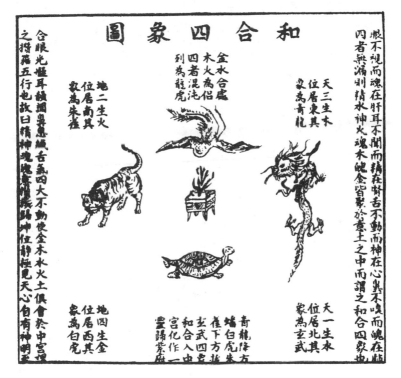

Interplay of Bird and Turtle

SOURCE: *Hsin Ming Kuei Ch'i*, vol. I, p. 17.

fighting, the bird flew back to the tree and the snake slithered back to the hole. The next day the whole scene was repeated. It was from observing this activity that Chang San-feng invented T'ai Chi Ch'uan. One of my teachers, an enlightened Taoist, told me that the bird represents the heart and the turtle represents the kidney; their fight symbolizes the interplay of heart and kidney. Thus Chang San-feng invented the T'ai Chi Ch'uan exercises to help achieve the purpose of meditation.

In my years of research into the relationship between T'ai Chi Ch'uan and meditation, I have found that the many movements of T'ai Chi Ch'uan facilitate the flow of *ch'i* through the body. The sequence of the form and meditation are almost the same. For example, in meditation the circulation of *ch'i* starts small with the Lesser Heavenly Circulation. It gradually develops to become the Greater Heavenly Circulation. Let us look first at the Beginning of the T'ai Chi Ch'uan form, which relates to the Lesser Heavenly Circulation of meditation.

Before starting, stand and relax while clearing the mind of all thoughts. Then you will be ready to start the exercise with the first form, the Beginning of T'ai Chi Ch'uan. As you stand erect with arms hanging loosely at sides and knees slightly bent (Figure 1), slowly breathe in and raise the hands to shoulder level (Figure 2). As you exhale, slowly lower the hands to the original position and bend the knees a little more, always keeping the spine erect. This movement of the arms raises the *ch'i* from its original position in the *tan-t'ien* up to the navel and back down to the *tan-t'ien*. In the terminology of meditation, this process is sometimes called the union of K'an and Li. K'an, representing water and the kidneys, also refers to the region of the lower abdomen, where the *tan-t'ien* is located. Li, which represents fire and the heart, designates the heart center. Thus the Beginning of T'ai Chi Ch'uan circulates the *ch'i* between these two vital centers. (In meditation the air (postnatal breathing) comes into the nostrils and sinks down to the navel. The *ch'i* (prenatal breathing) comes from the *tan-t'ien* and rises to the navel.) You may wish to repeat this movement several times before continuing on to Grasp Bird's Tail, which stabilizes the *ch'i* in the *tan-t'ien* as the right hand passes downward alongside the body (Figure 3). When the *ch'i* has stabilized, both the mind and breath are concentrated in the abdomen. In Taoist terminology this is referred to as Fire Dwells in the Water Place. Thus the abdomen is called a stove in meditation and has the capability of boiling the water, which is abundant in this place, to make steam. This diminishes the water and increases energy. It can prevent many illnesses and is also an integral part of the refinement of *ching* (sexual energy) into *ch'i* (energy). Hexagram 63 of the *I ching,* Wei Chi (After Completion) represents this image of fire below the water. A modern example for this image is the steam generator.

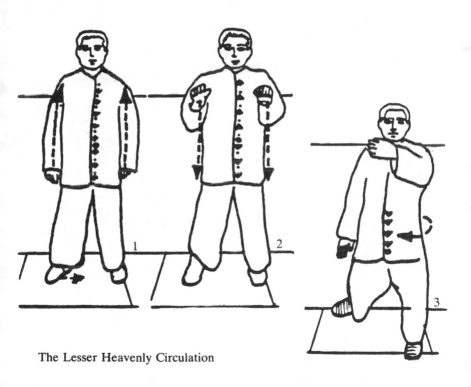

The Lesser Heavenly Circulation

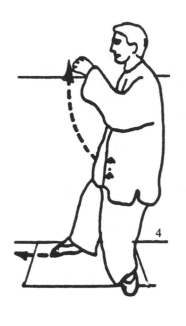

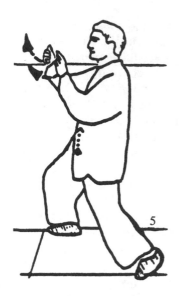

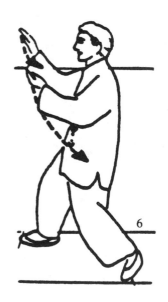

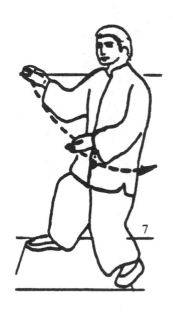

The next sequence begins with Push Up and continues to move the *ch'i* in the Lesser Heavenly Circulation. Turn to the right (Figure 4), and then move the right hand straight up in front of the body, bringing the *ch'i* from the abdomen to the navel (Figure 5). Then execute Pull Back (Figures 6 and 7), concentrating your mind and breathing on the motion of the left hand, which guides the *ch'i* from the navel back to the abdomen. The left hand circles around (Figure 8) and meets the right, palm to palm, at chest level (Figure 9). This posture is called Press Forward and again guides the *ch'i* from the abdomen to the navel. Now sit back and separate your hands (Figure 10), the *ch'i* returns to the abdomen by following the

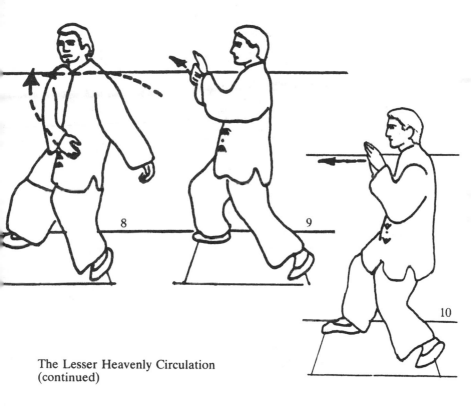

The Lesser Heavenly Circulation
(continued)

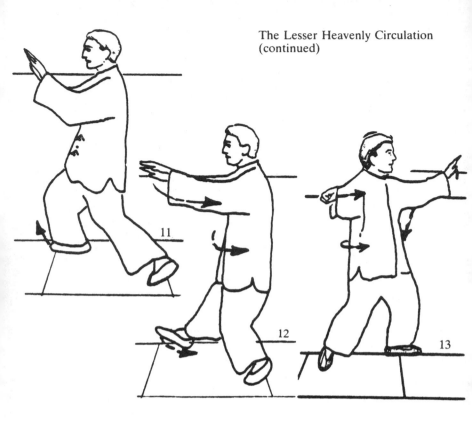

motion of the body as it sits back. The next posture is Push Forward (Figure 11), which sends the *ch'i* once more to the navel. This sequence is called Push Up, Pull Back, Press Forward, and Single Whip (PPPS for short). You may repeat PPPS one or more times from Push Up or even from the Beginning to achieve the Lesser Heavenly Circulation. Then you may continue with Turn Body and Single Whip (Figures 12 and 13). "Turn Body" means the turning point to begin a new process—the Greater Heavenly Circulation.

This process begins after the Single Whip when you extend your arms to each side, forming a half circle (Figure 14). The right leg is extended toward the corner, and in this open position the *ch'i* penetrates to the whole body. With the weight balanced over the left leg, you move both arms and the right leg toward the center in the form Play Guitar (Figure 15). The left palm is opposite the right elbow and the right leg rests lightly on the heel. The *ch'i* becomes concentrated along the Jen Mo. In the second section of the T'ai Chi Ch'uan form this same movement of *ch'i*—first opening and spreading to the whole body and then closing and concentrating along the Jen Mo—is achieved in the postures Slant Flying (Figure 25) and Play Guitar.

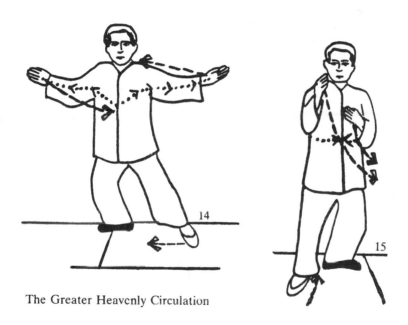

The Greater Heavenly Circulation

The sequence of forms continues after Play Guitar with Pull Back (Figure 16) and Step Forward and Strike with Shoulder (Figure 17), which constitute a conjunction joining the Lesser and Greater Heavenly Circulations. The Greater Heavenly Circulation actually begins with the form White Crane Spreads

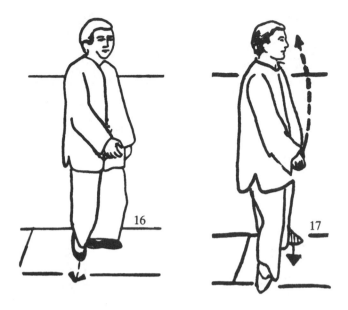

Wings (Figure 18). In this form the weight is balanced on the right foot and the right hand moves up to the front of the head. This upward movement of the hand guides the *ch'i* from the lower abdomen to the forehead, along the Jen Mo. As the form continues, the right knee bends lower, the right hand drops, and the trunk of the body rotates to the right (Figure 19). These coordinated movements guide the *ch'i* downward again along the Jen Mo from the forehead down to the lower abdomen. Then, nearly at the end of the rotation to the right, the right hand moves slightly behind the back. The purpose of this movement is to guide the *ch'i* from the lower abdomen through the pubic region and back to the base of the spine. The sequence continues with a step of the left foot, and then, as weight is shifted to the left, the left arm brushes past the left knee and the right arm circles back and around, passing by the ear to push forward. This form, called Brush Knee and Push Forward, guides the *ch'i* up the Tu Mo from the base of the spine along the spinal column to the crown of the head (Figure

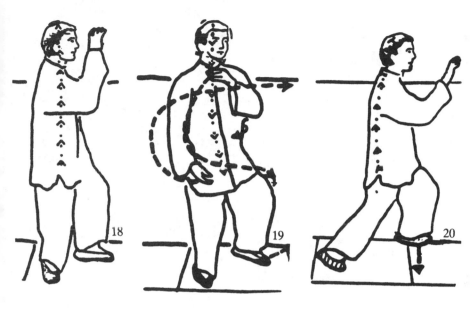

The Greater Heavenly Circulation (continued)

20). This movement is repeated three times in the short form and five times in the long form, alternating left and right. In fact, it can be repeated any odd number of times.

In T'ai Chi Ch'uan there are several postures that create a transition from section one to section two. For the purpose of meditation one may go directly from Brush Knee and Push Forward to Step Back and Repulse Monkey. In this posture the movement of the *ch'i* is described by this movement of your hands. The right hand drops to the region of the thigh, moves back and rises to the top of the head, and then is pushed forward and down, returning to the starting point. The left hand describes the same movement (Figures 21–23). However, when the right hand is at the top of the head, the left hand is in the thigh region. The relation of the two hands can be thought of as two diametrically opposed spokes of a wheel, while the movement of the wheel itself signifies the orbiting of the *ch'i* through the Greater Heavenly Circulation. This form may be repeated three, five, or seven times and may alternate

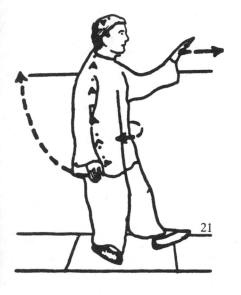

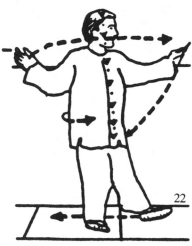

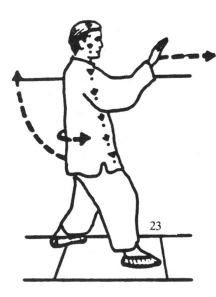

The Greater Heavenly Circulation
(continued)

with Brush Knee and Push Forward. The sequence of forms
we have just described is especially designed to guide the upward and downward flow as well as the forward and backward
flow of the *ch'i*.

After the last repetition of Step Back and Repulse Monkey,
drop the right hand to the left thigh and let the left hand circle
around and rest on the right wrist (Figure 24). Turn your body
to the right as you take a large step with the right foot and
transfer your weight onto it. Simultaneously the right hand,
with the palm up, moves diagonally across the front of the
body, resembling a bird's flight along a river bank, and lands
at the level of the temple. The left hand brushes the left knee
and comes to rest at the left side. This movement, called Slant
Flying, opens the whole body and allows the *ch'i* to penetrate
to every part of the body (Figure 25).

Now move the left foot up and transfer most of your
weight onto it. Simultaneously both arms and the right leg
move toward the center, taking the form Play Guitar (Figure
15). The left hand is opposite the right elbow and the right

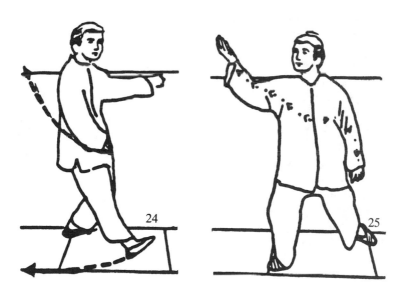

24

25

foot rests on its heel. By this motion the *ch'i* has become concentrated along the Jen Mo. In the next form, Pull Back, the arms and right leg retreat (Figure 16) and the *ch'i* moves down to the abdomen. As you perform Step Forward and Strike with Shoulder (Figure 17), the weight of the body shifts to the right foot and the *ch'i* sinks down to the Mortal Gate, or perineum.

White Crane Spreads Wings is the next posture in the sequence. It is the second time it occurs, and here it is the core of the form—the actual achievement of the Greater Heavenly Circulation. The entire weight is on the right foot, while the left foot moves to the center and rests lightly on the toes (Figure 18). Simultaneously, the right hand, palm downward, rises straight up to the forehead. These motions, combined with the concentration of the mind, raise the *ch'i* from the Mortal Gate, through the abdomen and the heart, to the top of the head (*ni-wan*). This is negative motion along the Jen Mo. The eyes look up as if to see through the top of the head. One imagines the total concentration of the mind and *ch'i* at *ni-wan*. The eyes are very important in meditation, as they represent the mind and guide the *ch'i* through the body.[2] The eyes are also important in T'ai Chi Ch'uan. T'ai Chi masters always advise that when your eyes see a point in space, the mind can reach this place and the hand and *ch'i* will follow to the same place.

As the form continues, the right hand turns over and drops down to the right side while the left hand rises in front of the body. The two palms are opposite each other as if holding a large ball (Figure 19). With this movement the mind, breathing and *ch'i* descend to the Mortal Gate along the Jen Mo, this time in a positive direction.

As before, Brush Knee and Push Forward is the next position. The right hand moves backward, bringing the *ch'i* from the Mortal Gate to the tip of the spinal cord. The right hand continues back, turns, and rises to describe a large circle, which passes by the ear to the front of the body. The left hand brushes the left knee (Figure 20). Both imagination and physical movement have led the *ch'i* upward from the tip of the spinal cord to the top of the head in positive motion along the Tu Mo.

Now you move the right foot up and center your weight over it. The left hand rests on the right arm and the whole body lowers, bending at the knees (Figure 26). This position is called Needle at Sea Bottom. The needle indicates the *ch'i* and the sea bottom is the lower part of the abdomen, or *ch'i-hai,* the Sea of Breath. The eyes are focused on the tip of the fingers of the right hand, and thus the *ch'i* moves from the top of the head down along the Jen Mo to the Mortal Gate. This motion along the Jen Mo completes the positive Greater Heavenly Circulation for meditation.

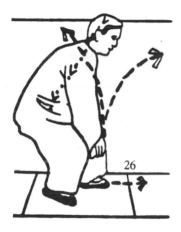

The Greater Heavenly Circulation (continued)

Now raise your body and step forward with the left foot, opening the arms in Play Arms Like a Fan (Figure 27). The right hand causes the *ch'i* to rise from *ch'i-hai* to the head in a negative direction along the Jen Mo, and the eyes and the mind once again concentrate on *ni-wan.* Now you throw your

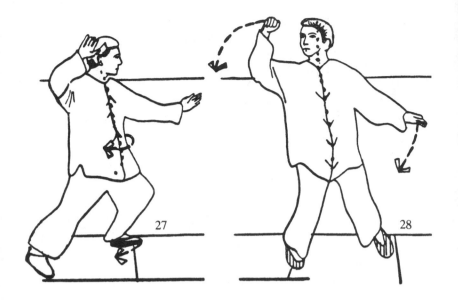

27   28

fist to the back of your head (Figure 28). The eyes follow the
course of the energy down through the head to the back, and
the *ch'i* follows the fist down the back to the tip of the spine.
This is negative motion along the Tu Mo, thus completing the
negative Greater Heavenly Circulation. The *ch'i* is now concentrated at the tip of the spine. The body completes this turn
to the back (Figure 29), and the *ch'i* makes a small circle in the
Mortal Gate. You step forward with the left foot and punch
(Figure 30). This brings the *ch'i* from the Mortal Gate to
ch'i-hai. Now pull back to the right side, bringing the *ch'i* back
to the Mortal Gate. Step forward with the right foot, raising
the hands in Push Up (Figure 5). The *ch'i* moves from the
Mortal Gate, through *ch'i-hai* and *tan-t'ien,* to the heart
center. Now perform Pull Back (Figures 6 and 7), with the
arms and the weight to the left side, bringing the *ch'i* back to
the Mortal Gate. Then perform Press Forward, the hands at
chest level guiding the *ch'i* back to the heart center (Figures 8
and 9). Sit back and separate your hands (Figure 10), and the

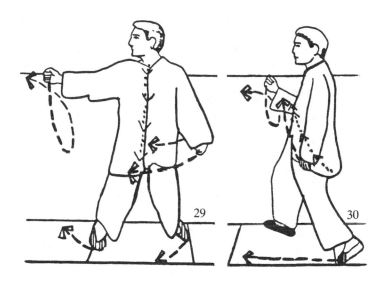

The Greater Heavenly Circulation (continued)

ch'i returns to the Mortal Gate. Perform Push Forward (Figure 11), and the *ch'i* once again moves forward and up to the heart. Now sit back, bringing the *ch'i* back to the Mortal Gate. At this point you may repeat the sequence one or more times from White Crane Spreads Wings to achieve the Greater Heavenly Circulation for meditation. After the last repetition of Push Forward, execute Turn Body to the Single Whip (Turn Body and Kick in the short form) and begin a new process with Wave Hands Like Clouds to achieve Turning the Wheel of Law from Left to Right and Reverse.

Many meditators are acquainted with the Greater Heavenly Circulation from front to back and back to front. This is called Turning the Wheel of Law from Back to Front and Reverse. However, only a few know about Turning the Wheel of Law from Left to Right and Reverse. It is pictured and described in *Hsin Ming Kuei Ch'i* (see illustration) and makes use of Wave Hands Like a Cloud. In this posture the left hand moves from the lower left side of the abdomen, across the body to the right

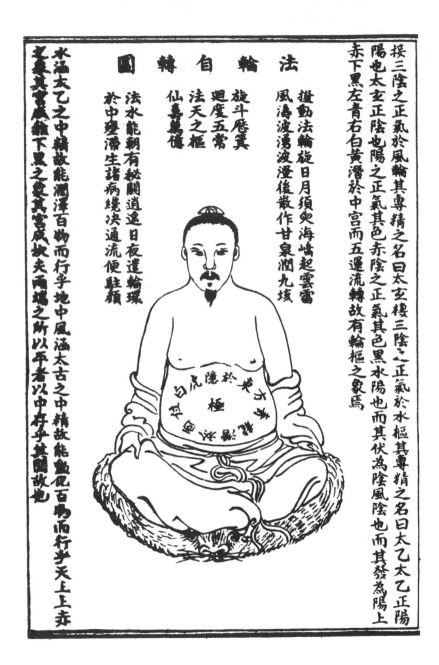

Turning the Wheel of Law from Left to Right and Reverse

SOURCE: *Hsin Ming Kuei Ch'i,* vol. 2, p. 12.

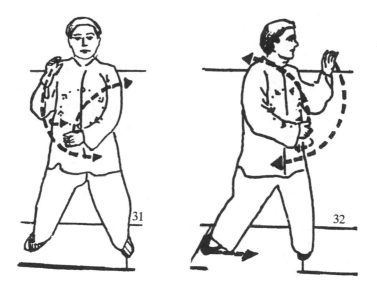

Turning the Wheel of Law from Left to Right and Reverse

side, up to the chest and back across the body to the left and down again as you step to the left (Figure 31). Then move your right foot close to the left and shift your weight onto it. The right hand performs a movement opposite to the left, starting at the lower right side of the abdomen, crossing the body to the left side, up to the chest, and back across the body to the right and down again (Figure 32). The motion of the arms traces the shape of a wheel in the air, which induces the *ch'i* to move in the shape of a wheel inside the body—achieving Turning the Wheel of Law from Left to Right and Reverse. This movement continues as long as time and space permit. When the player can no longer move to the left, he can reverse directions and move to the right. If space is extremely limited, this movement can be done from a fixed position, concentrating the mind and moving just the arms from left to right. It is very effective when performed in the fresh air but can be done anywhere, even in an office.

Now you have achieved both the Greater Heavenly Circulation and Turning the Wheel of Law from Left to Right and Reverse. These two circulations are the framework for the Mao Yu Circulation which moves the *ch'i* to every part of the body as the planets move in their orbits (see illustration). In meditation this is the most advanced level, and the corresponding form in T'ai Chi Ch'uan is Fair Lady Works at Shuttle, which comes in the last part of the exercise. The name Fair Lady Works at Shuttle describes the movements themselves, in which one turns successively to the left, to the right, and then to the left and the right once again, resembling the backward and forward and left and right movements of a shuttle. The succession of turns and pivots that comprise the movements of this form can be used to guide the *ch'i* in a circulation that passes diagonally through the trunk of the body. Commencing these movements from the end of the Single Whip, one first turns to the right, pivoting on the right heel and moving the left hand down in front of the belly, palm upward. This guides the *ch'i* downward and concentrates it on the right side of the lower abdomen. Then, after the small step with the right foot and the step to the northeast corner with the left foot, the weight shifts to the left, the body turning at the waist, while at the same time the left hand moves up to the left (Figure 33). This combination of movements send the *ch'i* upward diagonally across the front of the body to the left shoulder. After this has been done, the weight shifts to the right, and there is a right turn pivoting on the left heel, followed by a large step to the right (Figure 34). During this turn and step, the left hand lowers below the shoulder and the right hand drops across the front of the body, guiding the *ch'i* downward diagonally to the right lower abdomen and then around the right lower back. As the body turns farther to the right after the large step with the right foot, the *ch'i* shifts across the left side of the back. As weight shifts to the right, accompanied by the right turn at the waist, the raising of the right hand to the forehead, and the left palm pushing diagonally forward to the right, the *ch'i* is sent diagonally across the back upward to the right shoulder (Figure 35).

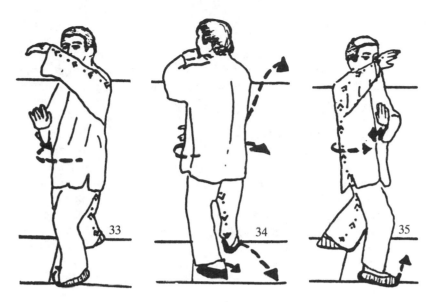

The Mao Yu Circulation

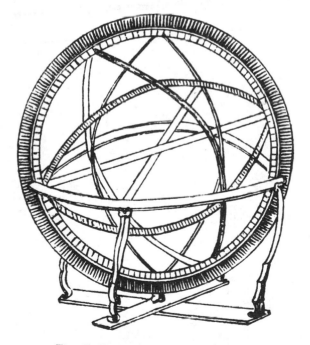

The Palindrome

SOURCE: *Hsin Ming Kuei Ch'i*, vol. 3, p. 11.

The remaining movements of the Fair Lady Works at Shuttle repeat this circulation once again. After the step to the southwest corner with the left foot, the *ch'i* is guided diagonally across the front to the left shoulder (Figure 36). Then, during the turn to the right, it is sent first down to the right lower abdomen, then around to the back (Figure 37), across to the left side of the back, and then diagonally over the back to the right shoulder once again (Figure 38). The diagonal circulation of the *ch'i* which is developed by this form is described in the *Hsin Ming Kuei Ch'i* as Palindromic Circulation, a reference to an ancient Chinese astronomical instrument which represents the orbits of the stars and planets in the heavens.

The circulation just described can be referred to as the Orbit of Inner Space as the *ch'i* circles through the torso. The Mao Yu Circulation can also be extended to the feet and fingers, in

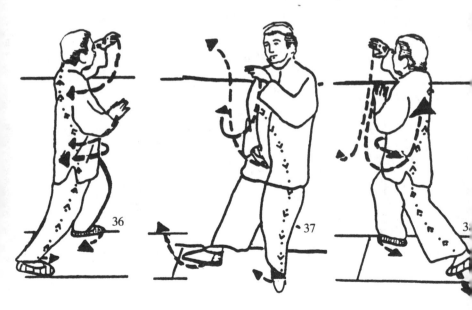

which case it is called the Orbit of Outer Space. This may be described as follows.

1. Beginning again from the Single Whip, the *ch'i* follows the left hand to the right side of the lower abdomen as you pivot on the right heel. Turning the right toes sends the *ch'i* to the back, and it drops down to the right foot as the weight is transferred to it. Then, as you step to the corner with the left foot and shift your weight onto it, the left hand moves up to the forehead and the right hand pushes diagonally forward to the left. During these motions the *ch'i* ascends from the right foot, through the leg, and crosses the back diagonally to the left shoulder, through the arm to the fingertips (Figure 33).

2. From this position you pivot on the left foot, lowering the left arm. The *ch'i* follows the left arm to the lower right side of the abdomen. As you pivot on the toes of the right foot, the *ch'i* circles to the back of the body, and as you transfer weight to the left foot, the *ch'i* descends to it (Figure 34). Now you step to the corner on the right foot, raising the *ch'i* to the lower back as your right arm reaches the forehead. Then, as you push forward diagonally to the right with the left hand, the *ch'i* crosses the back diagonally to the right shoulder along the arm to the fingers (Figure 35).

3. As you pull back the left arm, the *ch'i* descends to the left side of the lower abdomen, and as you step to the left with the right foot, the *ch'i* circles to the back. As you shift all your weight to the right foot, the *ch'i* descends to it. Now you step to the corner with the left foot, raising the *ch'i* to the lower back as your left arm reaches your forehead. Then, as you push forward diagonally to the left with the right hand, the *ch'i* crosses the back diagonally to the left shoulder through the arm to the fingertips (Figure 36).

4. The *ch'i* follows the right arm down to the right side of the lower abdomen as you pivot on your left foot. The *ch'i*

circles to the back as you pivot on your heel (Figure 37).
Shifting the weight to the left foot brings the *ch'i* down to it.
Then, as you step to the corner on your right foot and raise
your right arm to your forehead, the *ch'i* ascends through the
left leg. Finally, as you push forward diagonally to the right
with the left hand, the *ch'i* crosses the back diagonally to the
right shoulder, along the arm to the fingers (Figure 38).

Grasp Bird's Tail follows, and it centralizes the *ch'i* in the
abdomen once again. The PPPS sequence follows Grasp Bird's
Tail and provides the connection that allows you to perform
Fair Lady Works at Shuttle as many times as you wish. After
the last Single Whip, you may continue to Snake Creeps Down,
Step Forward, Seven Stars, Ride Tiger to the Mountain, and
Turn Body and Do Lotus Kick. In performing the turn, the
right leg acts as an axis and the left hand acts as a wheel, which
guides both the *ch'i* and the body (Figures 39–40). The *ch'i*
circles about the waist, and the body makes a revolution
through 360 degrees. This is a cycle through a horizontal plane
and completes the whole Mao Yu Circulation.

It is worth emphasizing that the T'ai Chi Ch'uan form en-
courages the flow of the *ch'i* to every part of the body, not
merely in the channels of control and function and to the left
and right of the belly. A useful analogy might be that of the
flow of traffic through the countryside: much of it travels on
major highways, but it extends to the back roads as well.
Nevertheless, it is very useful, particularly when one is learning to perceive the flow through the psychic channels, to perform repeatedly those parts of the exercise that encourage
circulation of a particular kind. To do this, instead of performing the entire sequence of movements in the usual order, you
can combine a few movements in a repeating cycle. There are
ways to do this easily, even if you have limited space. For
example, the Greater Heavenly Circulation can be repeated by
going through the Brush Knee and Push Forward, first with
the right, then with the left, and so on. When there is no room
left, it can be continued by changing to Step Back and Repulse

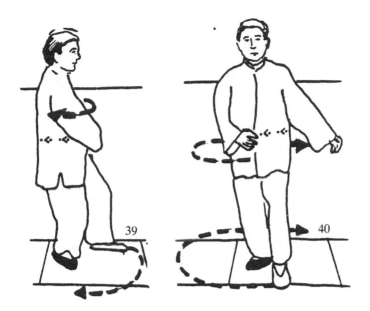

Circulation Through a Horizontal Plane

Monkey. When there is no more room to step back, you begin to Brush Knee and Push Forward once again. For the left-to-right circulation, Wave Hands Like Clouds can be performed as a cycle if you simply begin to step to the right after there is no more room to step to the left. And for the Mao Yu Circulation, it is obvious that Fair Lady Works at Shuttle can be repeated indefinitely without exceeding the limits of a rather small square.

It is necessary to understand that the roles of the mind and the *ch'i* are even more important than the movements themselves. The *Classics of T'ai Chi Ch'uan* say: "The mind directs the *ch'i* and the *ch'i* mobilizes the body." The mind indeed guides the *ch'i* to every part of the body, including the smallest cavities and the bones. During certain movements the *ch'i* may have several destinations. For example, in Fair Lady Works at Shuttle, the *ch'i* may circulate through and around the torso, or the mind may direct the *ch'i* all the way to the fingers and toes. While the outer movements remain the same, the inner movements of *ch'i* have gone farther and deeper. The mind also directs the breathing, which is very important to both T'ai Chi Ch'uan and meditation practice, for the outside breath is one element of the formation of *ch'i* (energy). I have not mentioned the breathing in the above descriptions of the form to avoid confusing the reader.

I include the picture of the movements of T'ai Chi Ch'uan, which indicate the relation between the outside movements coordinated with breathing or *ch'i* inside. The arrows with short broken lines indicate the movements outside. The arrowheads as darts point out the direction of the *ch'i* upward, downward, left or right. This shows that the movements and the *ch'i* or breathing have a close relation. Not only does the *ch'i* pilot the movements, but the movements help the *ch'i* flowing inside. The reader can achieve this purpose easily.

NOTES

1. The snake symbolizes man while the turtle symbolizes woman. These symbols are interchangeable in the illustrations that appear of this story.
2. This process is described in detail in Lu K'uan Yu, *Taoist Yoga*, pp. 62–64.

CHAPTER ELEVEN

DAILY LIFE: SITTING, STANDING, WALKING, SLEEPING

The meditator's daily life is no different from that of other people—he or she sits, stands, walks, and sleeps just as they do. However, the meditator uses these actions to help achieve the goals of meditation. To Meditative Sitting, Meditative Standing, Meditative Walking, and Meditative Sleeping, the more advanced add a form called Meditative Squatting.[1]

MEDITATIVE SITTING

There are two kinds of sitting. One is for the purpose of rest. For this, you may sit in any position that you find comfortable. More important than posture here is a serene mind, free from anxious thoughts. Direct the mind and the breathing to the *tan-t'ien* or abdomen in order to feel restful.

The second kind of sitting is Meditative Sitting. It affects many neural meridians, from the feet to such areas of the upper body as the kidneys, liver, and spleen. The heat created by this exercise increases blood circulation and helps the stomach digest food. Rheumatism and arthritis can be cured and prevented by this method.

In Meditative Sitting, correct posture is very important. After you have finished eating, sit erect in a chair of sensible height, enabling the feet to rest comfortably on the floor. Direct the mind and the breathing to the *tan-t'ien* and place the tongue against the palate to gather saliva. When swallowed, the saliva reproduces the vitality or sexual essence. Cover your knees with the palms of your hands, with your fingers against the indentations at the bases of the kneecaps. Exert a light pressure with the middle three fingers of each hand. Press the ring finger of each hand against the outer hollow (called *tu-pi* or Calf's Nose), the middle finger against the central cavity (*shih-shia*), and the index finger against the inner joint (the *shih-yen* or Eyes of the Knees).

Meditative Sitting is convenient and easy to do. It can be performed anywhere, even when you are sitting in an office or in your bedroom before retiring at night. You may continue to apply pressure to the meridians in the knees as long as you like, to improve the circulation and help the inner organs of the abdomen function well.

MEDITATIVE STANDING

Many people stand with a bad posture, giving no thought to how this affects the spine and inner organs. Even when you are just standing for no particular purpose, you should observe certain practices. Keep the head erect and the spinal cord straight. Do not lean back, forward, or to the side. Direct the weight of your body to your legs instead of retaining a tightness in your shoulders. In sum, be as erect and as rooted as a pine tree.

Meditative Standing can be performed under various circumstances. It is best conducted in the fresh air and sunshine. The surroundings—trees and plants—will benefit you. In time, Meditative Standing can also give you the opportunity to master many methods of breathing.

The rays of the sun are beneficial to Meditative Standing. The Taoists believe that Yang, "Essence from Heaven," is transferred from the sunshine to the body. It is wise to practice Meditative Standing in the early hours of the morning when the air is fresher and cleaner. Even before sunrise, the sky is redder, thus more powerful. If possible, stand in the open air before the sun comes up in order to receive its energy through deep breathing. At noontime, benefit from the sun's rays by facing south. Inhale deeply into the abdomen and "swallow" your breath. In the evening, again face the sun and swallow the air you breathe in. Even at sunset, the sun's energy can be received from the last traces of yellow and red in the western sky.

In ancient times, the Taoists believed that sunlight only transmitted a spiritual essence from heaven. It has now been established that solar energy can be used to heat homes and power machines. Modern medical science has also concluded that solar energy combines with ultraviolet rays to make chemical changes in the body, thereby producing vitamin D, killing germs, and activating the production of sex hormones.

Another form of Meditative Standing takes advantage of the oxygen given off by vegetation. In Taoist teachings, the inner elixir was long ago likened to plants in that it sprouts, blossoms, and goes to seed. If one breathed deeply in front of trees and plants, the Taoists said, the essence from the plants was transferred to the meditator to replenish the energy of the body. Today, of course, we know as a scientific fact that plants provide oxygen, which cleans the blood circulating to the tissues of the body. Thus, the Taoists were correct when they recommended that one should stand in front of trees and plants, breathe deeply into the abdomen, and swallow the air. This form of Meditative Standing is most effective in the spring, when the trees spread their leaves and blossom.

Another practical advantage to Meditative Standing is that it can help the meditator practice various types of breathing. One breathing method is relatively simple. Stand erect with the feet at shoulder width. Place the palms of the hand against the abdomen, lean slightly forward with the torso, and breathe out through the nose to push out stale air. Now stand erect with hands at sides, and inhale fresh air through the nostrils, directing the mind and the breath to the abdomen. Exhale and inhale in this fashion for three completed breaths. It is best to perform this exercise in the morning.

If you practice Meditative Standing in quiet surroundings and with a peaceful mind, you can attempt a series of more sophisticated breathing techniques. Begin by inhaling the air deep into the abdomen for, say, a slow count of five; hold the breath there for another count of five; exhale the old air at the same speed. As you advance in skill, you can store the breath in the abdomen for a longer count than that of the inhaling and exhaling. Eventually the *tan-t'ien* will become warm. But storing the breathing must be done in a natural fashion, doing it with force or strain will cause harm.

More advanced meditators can use Meditative Standing to direct the *ch'i* to various parts of the body for cleansing purposes. First, increase the warmth in the abdomen by using the mind to direct the *ch'i* to the *tan-t'ien*. Now guide the *ch'i* and the mind from the *tan-t'ien* to your legs as you exhale; then guide them back to the abdomen as you inhale. This cleanses the front of your body. Also use the mind and the breathing to penetrate the back of the body. Continuing in this way, breathe in through the nostrils and slowly concentrate your mind to the neck and down to the lower back. When it reaches the lower back, breathe out and relax your mind a short while. Now inhale and slowly return your mind from the lower back, up to the head, and through the nostrils. This is one unit. Continue this procedure three, five, or seven times to clean and penetrate the Tu Mo, or Channel of Control.

Concentration of the mind and the *ch'i* can also clear the head. Breathe in through the nose and direct the thought and the breath up the crown and back to the medulla oblongata. Breathe out after it has reached the back of the head, using the mind to guide the *ch'i* back to the crown and out through the nose. Repeat this three, five, or seven times in order to improve concentration, cleanse the mind, and make it more peaceful. Meditative Standing in this fashion paves the way for the Sitting

Meditation cited earlier, which brings the vitality from the back
of the body or Tu Mo through the head to the front—completing the cycle of the Greater Heavenly Circulation.

MEDITATIVE WALKING

Everyday walking is different from Meditative Walking.
When you walk to your job, you may be subjected to pollution
and jarring crowds. Your mind is likely to be set with a purpose, a destination you feel you must reach quickly. But there
are proper ways to walk, even for common errands. Keep the
head and spinal cord erect. Direct the weight to the legs rather
then the shoulders and head. Plant the feet firmly on the
ground to establish good balance, and maintain a quiet, alert
mind. I have walked daily in such a fashion without falling for
more than twenty years.
· For Meditative Walking, it is good to walk in a garden. The
conditions are quiet, the air is cleaner than on the street, and
the surrounding plants increase the supply of oxygen. Concentrate the mind without tension. Cast the eyes forward and
place the tongue against the palate. Walk with the body erect,
the shoulders relaxed, and the elbow and knee joints loose.
Let the arms hang naturally at the sides, swinging neither too
high nor too low, in coordination with the step. As in T'ai Chi
Ch'uan, the fingers should not be separate but should curve
naturally. Direct the bulk of your weight to below the navel.
The foot touching the ground should bear the brunt of your
weight, while the other foot remains light and weightless.
Wear shoes that are roomy enough to let the toes and feet
move comfortably. Thus, when you place the whole bottom of
the foot on the ground while walking, the pressure of the step
stimulates the veins, arteries, nerve lines, and glands contained there.
Meditative Walking is auxiliary to Sitting Meditation. In
Sitting Meditation, you are isolated and silent; as stated in the

previous chapter, the beginner discovers that his mind tends to wander with anxious thoughts. However, Meditative Walking takes place in the fresh air and exercises every part of your body. As you walk, the mind, the *ch'i,* and the movement are coordinated. Blood circulates from the feet and legs throughout the whole body to maintain both physical and mental health. With the body and mind refreshed, it is easier for the beginner to assume the posture of Sitting Meditation and to concentrate with a clear mind.

MEDITATIVE SLEEPING

Sleep proves especially soothing for workers who undergo mental stress, fatigue, and a drain of energy at the job. Many people lose precious vitality because of insomnia and take pills in order to sleep; others lose energy from nocturnal emissions.

My *Taoist Health Exercise Book* describes two forms of sleep for health. In one method, the pillow is raised to facilitate breathing. Lie face up on a bed or the floor and cover the abdomen with your palms. When exhaling, press lightly with the hands to expel stale air; while inhaling, release this pressure. The movement resembles the action of a bellows, warming the *tan-t'ien* and helping the breathing. This should be done about ten times. The second method of sleep is used when you sleep on one side. Make certain that the pillow is neither too high nor too low. Rest the cheek of the side you are lying on against the open palm of your hand. Bend your knees slightly (with the upper leg a bit shorter than the lower one), and place your other hand comfortably along the upper thigh.

A more sophisticated practice is Meditative Sleeping. Like Sitting Meditation, it requires great skill and should only be attempted by accomplished Taoist masters. I include this material for your information, not to recommend its practice.

Some Taoist masters have tapped the vitality through Meditative Sleeping, as a means of attaining the goals of medita-

tion. For example, many Chinese books credit immortality to
Ch'en T'uan. They claim that, through meditation, he could
sleep for days and years at a time. And the life of Chang
San-feng is said to have spanned from the twelfth to the four-
teenth centuries—including the late Sung dynasty, the Yuan
dynasty, and the early Ming dynasty—because of meditation
and Meditative Sleeping. In their teachings and writings, the
Taoists did not detail the methods used by such masters to
perfect this form of meditation. For years, I thought they were
selfishly guarding a secret to longevity. But I have since come
to understand and appreciate the dangers involved and the
reasons for their reticence.

One of the most enlightened Taoists described to me the
Ch'en T'uan method of Meditative Sleeping as follows: When
the master sleeps on his right side, he cradles the right cheek
with the palm of his hand. He lightly presses his right thumb
against the cavity at the base of the ear. This crevice—where
the jaw meets the skull—is known in acupuncture as *yi-fung*.
The two legs are bent, with the left knee slightly above the
right. The master holds the upper calf of the left leg with his
left hand and lightly presses his thumb against the soft center
at the back of the knee. The light pressure of the thumbs at
these neural meridians benefits the kidneys, harmonizes the
inner organs, improves sleep, and helps achieve the inner
elixir. While drifting off to sleep, his mind contemplates the
"divine fetus" residing in the *tan-t'ien*.

In describing Ch'en T'uan's method of Meditative Sleeping,
the speaker included a sober warning. If one does it incor-
rectly or lacks a sufficiently peaceful mind, one can easily
succumb to danger. For example, when Ch'en T'uan's meditation had reached its highest level, he had stored enough sur-
plus energy to nourish and sustain his body for long periods of
sleep without ruin. This extended sleep is like meditation. It is
unlikely that the reader possesses such discipline and skill to
store such great amounts of energy and to use it while sleeping. In addition, disciples tended to Ch'en T'uan's every need,
protecting him from outside disturbances (such as noise and

weather) and waking him whenever necessary. Unless you can rely upon a guardian who will anticipate your needs and protect you continually for extended periods, this form should be avoided.

MEDITATIVE SQUATTING

Squatting has benefits for both health and meditation. Simple squatting, as mentioned in my *Taoist Health Exercise Book,* is healthful because it straightens the spine, harmonizes the breathing, and brings peace of mind. Meditative Squatting has long been performed by monks in the Buddhist temples of Burma. With their hands together at eye level, the monks appear to be praying. The form was also taught by Master Du. However, Meditative Squatting can be most perilous for the amateur. It can drive a person mad unless he has mastered a profound mental discipline of concentration and inner peace. I do not recommend that you attempt this exercise, which I describe for your interest only.

Yang Shen's book *Record of a 250-Year-Old-Man* (published in Chinese) contains Master Li Ch'ing Yuen's description of how he performed Meditative Squatting to cultivate fetal breathing. Li began in the posture of Sitting Meditation until he achieved the phenomenon of forgetting his surroundings and even himself. In this state, vitality stored in the *tan-t'ien* made inhaling and exhaling unncessary, and he stopped breathing. So dynamic was this vitality that his abdomen felt as hot as scalding water. At this point, Li squatted like a monkey to perform a series of breathing exercises. With his neck pulled back into his torso and his shoulders hunched up, the squatting meditator breathed from his heels. At the first stage, he breathed in this fashion twelve times, shrank the abdomen inward, and tightened the muscles of the anus. With his mind, he guided the scalding energy from the *tan-t'ien* to the base of the spine (*wei-lu*). Again he breathed twelve times from the heels, this time guiding the hot vitality from the abdomen to the middle of the spine—known as *chia-chi* or *chi-chung*. A third series of twelve breaths from the heels fanned the power in the abdomen, which was directed to the back of the skull, or *yu-chen*. The form climaxed with twenty-four breaths from the heels and nine blinks of the eyes. The blinking helped to bring the vitality from the *yu-chen* to the crown of the head (*ni-wan*). The powerful energy now traveled down the center of the forehead (*ming-t'ang*) through the nose to the mouth. With his tongue against his palate, this energy was collected as saliva, which, when swallowed, was returned to the abdomen. This was considered one cycle of current. Practiced without a confused mind for long periods of time, such Meditative Squatting has been said to result in longevity.

NOTE

1. For further details, see my *Taoist Health Exercise Book*, pp. 21–44, 63–64.

CHAPTER TWELVE

SEXUAL ENERGY: PRODUCTION, RETENTION, TRANSFORMATION, AND CIRCULATION

The Taoists believe that male and female are indispensable to each other. Sexuality not only is important to the maintenance of a healthy and happy life, but can also result ultimately in the achievement of longevity.

The emperor-sage Huang Ti, who wrote the first book of Chinese medical science, the *Nei ching,* also believed that sex was beneficial to health, according to the principles of yin and yang. He conducted many experiments with female assistants. Through this work he developed both the philosophical ideas and the postures used in sexual activity. These ideas were recorded in a book called the *Su nu ching,* or *"The Immaculate Girl's Book."* It takes the form of a dialogue between Huang Ti and his assistant/concubine, Su Nu. They discuss in great detail the correct forms for sexual activity and the benefits of proper performance of them. This book has been translated into Japanese as *Ishinho* and into English under the name *The Tao of Sex.* It is more detailed than most modern sexual books.

Later Taoist medical doctors and alchemists clarified and elaborated upon these ancient ideas. They proposed that sexual energy is a very important element in the achievement of longevity and immortality. They said if you raise the *ching* to the brain, you can achieve longevity. (In man *ching* is the sperm, and in woman it is the ovum and the menstrual fluid.) Joseph Needham refers to this technique in volume 2 of his book *Science and Civilization in China,* but he expresses doubt that the process is physically possible. Surely, for the common person it is not easy. One must study with experts and practice over time, just as a scientist must study a long time and perform experiments in the laboratory to achieve his or her aim.

Many Taoist books describe the technique of purifying the *ching,* which is transformed into *ch'i* and finally into *shen.* This, they say, results in long life and also maintains the appearance and vitality of youth. Moreover, the Taoists emphasized that one who does not have the ability to produce a baby cannot achieve immortality. Chan San-feng said that if the *ching* flows downward, it will become a baby; if it flows upward, it will produce immortality.

Confucius believed that the action between man and woman was the beginning of heaven and earth. In the *Chung-yung,* the *Doctrine of the Mean,* he states: "The way of the superior man may be found, in its simple elements, in the intercourse of common men and women, but in its utmost reaches, it shines brightly through heaven and earth."[1]

In his writing *Ta chuan,* the *Great Treatise* on the *I ching,* he equates the intercourse of heaven and earth with that between man and woman: "The Master said: Heaven and earth come together, and all things take shape and find form. Male and female mix their seed, and all creatures take shape and are born."[2] Moreover, the Image of Hexagram 11, T'ai, says: "Heaven and Earth unite: the image of Peace."[3] The hexagram T'ai, or Peace, means a time of harmony and flourishing of life forces. On the contrary, the image of hexagram 12, P'i, states: "Heaven and earth do not unite: The image of standstill."[4] Thus the hexagram P'i also means stagnation and decline.

The same ideas can be found in Buddhism, especially in the branch known as Tantrism, which emphasized the importance of the relationship between man and woman. It was believed that a god (or buddha) obtained divine energy by embracing his female partner, or *shakti*. In one of the most important Buddhist Tantric texts, the *Guhyasamaja Tantra* or *Tathagata-guhyaka,* we find ideas that parallel the Taoist interest in breathing and sexual activity. In Tantric theory the male quality is emptiness (*sunyata*) and the female quality is life and compassion (*karuna*). Unity (*advaya*) is achieved through the sexual act. Thus the union of the sexes is said to be of the essence of Tantrism.[5] Like Taoism, Tantrism encouraged women practitioners as well as men. They also materialized these ideas in bronze statues showing sexual union between the god and the goddess who is his female counterpart. These were very popular in Chinese Buddhist temples, and examples of them can be found in American museums such as the Museum of Natural History in New York City.

Both in Tantrism and Taoism an activity called Double Meditation is emphasized for man and woman together. In another practice, called Single Meditation, the experience of male and female takes place within the body of the single meditator. Sexual union is imagined to take place within his or her body, without any outside influence.

Some books of meditation give instructions for the man only. In the later Sung dynasty (A.D. 1200), Sun Pu Erh, wife of Ma Tan Yang, the greatest of the Seven Immortals of the Northern Taoist school, wrote about the importance of man and woman to each other in her poems. For women the process of meditation is basically the same as for men; only a few points are different. When they have achieved immortality, the breasts become smaller, and the menstrual fluid becomes white, as if the woman were pregnant. This change signifies movement toward immortality.

HOW TO PRODUCE SEXUAL ENERGY

We have already noted that according to the Taoists, when sexual energy is discharged in the usual way, it leads to the conception of a baby; when it is reversed, the goal of immortality can be achieved. Therefore, it is easier for young people to achieve the goal of meditation than for older people. If they are virgins, they can achieve this much sooner. Old people do not produce sexual energy and so cannot readily achieve the goal of meditation. Most people are aware that a primary purpose of meditation is health and longevity. However, they may feel that it is too late, for even though they have the desire to achieve this end, they do not have the ability.[6] By using the method of circulating the breath through the eight psychic channels as described in the chapters on Standing and Sitting Meditation, sexual energy can be produced even by older people.[7] In this way, the channels become unblocked and the flow of sexual energy is unimpeded.

The following describe other methods of producing this energy.

1. Sitting on the edge of a chair the height of your knee, with body erect and feet firmly planted on the floor, rest your hands, palms down, on your knees. Slowly lean your torso forward and then slowly rise up to an erect position. When you rise up, breathe in; when you lean forward, breathe out. Do this twelve times. Then reverse: breathe out when you rise up, and breathe in when you lean forward. In this way, you draw the energy from your feet and the marrow from your legs to the pubic region. Increase gradually to eighteen and then to twenty-four times. This exercise should be done every morning and evening with the window open to let in fresh air. A man who does this exercise should use his mind to direct the energy from the glans of the penis to the perineum.

2. Practice T'ai Chi Ch'uan. The first stage is to learn the form and do it correctly. The second stage is to use your mind to direct the *ch'i* throughout your body as you do the form. In the *Classics of T'ai Chi Ch'uan,* in a chapter called "Commentary on the Use of the Mind and Body to Practice Thirteen Movements of T'ai Chi Ch'uan," this passage appears:

> The mind [the will] directs the *ch'i,* the breath, letting it sink down [to the abdomen], thereby penetrating even to the bones.
> . . . The mind is primary, the body secondary. The abdomen is relaxed and the *ch'i* penetrates to the bones. The mind remains quiet and the body at ease.
> . . . The forward and backward movements guide the *ch'i* to the back and concentrate the energy in the spinal cord.

T'ai Chi Ch'uan practiced in this way is very effective. I practice it myself every day. You will feel your whole body becoming warm, especially in the pubic area. This warmth indicates that sexual energy is being produced.

Both T'ai Chi Ch'uan and the exercise described under paragraph 2 alone are concerned with gathering the vitality to become the marrow of the bones. Most people do not understand that the marrow is related to sexual energy. One who is strong and has sexual energy, also has strong legs. One who is sick, weak, old, and without sexual energy has weak legs. That is the reason so many old people fall and break their legs.

3. Sexual energy is also closely related to the brain. If a person has sexual energy, his or her mind is intelligent. When a person is old, sick, or weak, the memory is poor. Western science has recently confirmed this connection recognized by the ancients. This relationship between the brain and sexual energy has been described as follows:

> [Essential] nature is spiritual vitality in the heart that manifests through the two channels from the center of the brain. So when seeing is concentrated on the spot between the eyes, the light of [essential] nature manifests and will, after a long training, unite with [eternal] life to become one whole.[8]

I myself observed this principle in my own meditation, which I practice daily for forty or fifty minutes. After one or two months, my sexual energy became very strong, my mind became very clear, my memory very good. I was able to work without feeling tired. However, this energy was very difficult to retain. I felt the desire for a woman and had nocturnal emissions which caused me to lose my sexual energy many times. After this happened, I was determined to prevent its reoccurrence. Yet I continued to find myself unable to control the emissions or my desires once my sexual energy reached its highest point as a result of meditation. As a result, I decided to use the ancient technique of Double Meditation, in which man and woman meditate together. I began to meditate with a female partner, but after a short time she discontinued our practice. I failed again. It is preferable to have a permanent partner.

4. Anyone can produce sexual energy by looking at erotic pictures or through contact (such as dancing) with someone of the opposite sex. When desire has been stimulated, there are several techniques that can be used to retain sexual energy.

You can concentrate on the cavity between life and death (between the anus and genitals) and contract the anus inward. Once you have mastered the technique, you can use your mind to transform sexual energy into vitality and draw this vitality up the spinal column to the head. Lui Tung Pin, who lived in the T'ang dynasty, was one of many Taoist immortals who practiced this technique. He spent a lot of time drinking and carousing with women. There is a legend that he once seduced a very beautiful young girl named White Peony. Another Taoist immortal from the Sung dynasty, Liu Hai Ch'an who spent a lot of time in brothels, became a Patriarch of the Southern Taoist school. He abstained from intercourse; when sexually aroused, he moved his energy up. There are two kinds of intercourse—the physical and the spiritual.

For the average person, deep breathing and concentration of

the mind can be used to retain sexual energy, and the following exercises can be practiced to distribute this energy throughout the body.

• Concentrate on the pubic area while doing the T'ai Chi Ch'uan movements White Crane Spreads Wing, Wave Hands Like Clouds, and Step Back and Repulse Monkey.

• If it is not convenient to do these movements, try this exercise: Hold your arms open as though you were holding a large ball, and slowly open and close your arms like bellows. When you open, breathe in, when you close your arms, breathe out. As you do this, concentrate on the pubic area. This exercise may seem too simple to be effective. However, it is basic to T'ai Chi Ch'uan and is derived from an ancient principle described in the *I ching:* " . . . they called the closing of the gates the Receptive, and the opening of the gate the Creative."[9] These exercises are very effective not only for preventing emission, but also for helping to produce sexual energy.

HOW TO RETAIN SEXUAL ENERGY

If it is difficult to produce sexual energy, it is more difficult to retain it. Even Taoist masters have lost their sexual energy, which they referred to as *lu-tan,* or "leaking the elixir." Many Taoist meditators sit day and night and avoid sleeping for fear of losing their sexual energy. Some use a special device to prevent emission.

A man may lose sexual energy for any of several reasons. Accidental physical contact with women is one example. The story is told of a Buddhist monk who was visited by a beautiful young woman. She knelt before him, and as she started to rise, she touched his leg to support herself. At her touch, the monk had an emission. Another example, according to my own experience, occurs during sleep. If the temperature is low and your body is well covered but during the night the temperature rises, an emission will occur. In winter, the reverse occurs—a drop of temperature during the night will have the same result. When the temperature is low and you sleep with your legs drawn up, the pressure of this position on the genital area can also bring on emission. Finally, I have found that when one is overtired and sleeps very deeply, emission will occur. The story is told in *Taoist Yoga* that the prize student of a Taoist master reported having lost his sexual energy from taking care of family affairs.

There are several methods to prevent such loss:

1. Do not become overexcited when in the presence of the opposite sex. Keep your mind quiet. Avoid reading love stories, looking at pornographic materials, or talking about sex before sleep. Do not think about past or present romances before falling asleep. Instead, read Taoist books.

2. If certain changes in temperature conditions are expected during the night, prepare your blanket accordingly. Before falling asleep, do not overeat. Your stomach should be somewhat empty.

3. Arrange your work schedule so that it is not too heavy, especially in the afternoon. Avoid strenuous exercise. In the evening, take a leisurely walk or do gentle exercises. Meditate regularly before sleep to relax your mind. If you are already able to transform sexual energy into *ch'i*, practice the circulation of the *ch'i* through the body several times. In Taoist terminology this is called "turning the water wheel." If you are a beginner, use deep breathing and the exercises described on page 135 to disperse the sexual energy.

TRANSFORMATION OF SEXUAL ENERGY

The whole process of meditation is one of transformation, an alchemical process. In the first step of this process, the elements of the inner organs are combined to produce sperm or egg cells. Just as the buried carcasses of animals after thousands of years become crude oil, which in turn is purified and becomes gasoline, so food becomes energy.

Chuang Tzu likened the next stage of the transformation of sexual energy to the process in which a fish from the Northern Ocean metamorphizes into a bird.[10] The Northern Ocean represents the abdomen, which is the region of water.

Confucius in his *Doctrine of the Golden Mean* also describes this process of transformation. Speaking of sincerity or concentration as the necessary attitude to achieve transformation, he says: " . . . This sincerity becomes apparent. From being apparent, it becomes manifest. From being manifest, it becomes brilliant. Brilliant, it affects others [moves]. Affecting [moving] others, they are changed by it. Changed by it, they are transformed."[11]

Concentration and sincerity are essential for meditation. In order to achieve enlightenment and transformation, the mind must direct the whole procedure from the perineum into the *tan-t'ien* or lower abdomen. That part of the body, known as the cauldron, becomes warm in meditation, as if it were plugged into a source of electric current. Warmth alone, however, is not enough to bring about the transformation. Wind, or breath, is needed to increase and intensify the heat. It takes a long time to achieve this stage of transformation of sexual energy into *ch'i*.

Meditation must continue without stopping, depending on the individual. Confucius says of this aspect of the process: " . . . to entire sincerity there belongs ceaselessness . . . not ceasing, it continues long. Continuing long, it evidences itself. Evidencing itself, it reaches far. Reaching far, it becomes large and substantial, it becomes high and brilliant."[12] Thus, with sincerity and continuous practice, sexual energy can be transformed into *ch'i*. Once this has happened, the *ch'i* must then be circulated by way of the spinal column throughout the whole body, just as gasoline must reach the engine in order for the car to move.

Commenting on the Taoist procedure of sending sexual energy to the brain, Joseph Needham wrote that it is impossible for sperm to reach the brain and be retained there. Actually, it is not the sperm or the egg cells themselves that are sent to the brain, but the *ch'i* into which these cells have been transformed through meditation.

CIRCULATION OF SEXUAL ENERGY

T'ai Chi Ch'uan and meditation are both systematic procedures for producing, transforming, and circulating sexual energy. Since this whole process requires continuous change, the practice of these disciplines must be regular and uninterrupted. If sexual energy is not transformed into *ch'i,* it cannot be retained. Just as water in a glass will overflow when it becomes too full, so sexual energy becomes a liquid (semen or menstrual flow) that will flow out. However, when it is transformed into *ch'i,* it becomes an inner force. However, this process can be compared to boiling water, which produces steam. If the steam is not directed into pipes, it will evaporate; or, when water boils and the cover of the pot is not removed, the force of the steam will knock the cover off. However, just as steam reverts to liquid when water ceases to boil, so the *ch'i* becomes sperm again if practice does not continue. Thus the *ch'i* must be transformed into *shen* in order to achieve the highest goal of meditation.

The techniques involved in both the T'ai Chi Ch'uan and meditation require that the mind and breath work together according to a prescribed procedure. In meditation, this procedure consists of letting the mind guide the circulation breath to certain centers of the body through a series of channels or pathways connecting these centers. The circulation or transformation process goes through two phases. In the first stage, the mind directs the *ch'i* or breath from the lung and heart area to the genital and kidney area and back again to the heart. This is called the Lesser Heavenly Circulation. In the second stage, the Greater Heavenly Circulation, the *ch'i* is directed from the genital region to the base of the spine and up the spinal column to the top of the head, where it is transformed into *shen*. *Shen* is then transformed into *shu*, or emptiness. *Shu* is directed from the top of the head, down into the throat, where it becomes saliva, and finally down the chest into the abdomen.

The path of the Greater Heavenly Circulation is analogous to the passage of the four seasons of the year. From the abdomen to the spine is spring; from the spine to the top of the head is summer; from the top of the head to the chest is autumn; and from the chest to the abdomen is winter. In Taoist writings the Greater Circulation is often referred to as 360 days. The Lesser Circulation is comparable to a whole day. The heart is the sun and the liver the moon.

The procedure described above relates to meditation. The movements of T'ai Chi Ch'uan also stimulate this process.

The T'ai Chi Ch'uan classic called the *Song of the Thirteen Movements* says: "When the lower spine is erect, the *ch'i*-vitality will reach the top of the head [Tu Mo—channel of control]." The T'ai Chi Treatise says: "When the neck is erect, use your mind to direct the *ch'i* to the top of the head, then sinking down to the abdomen (*tan-t'ien*) [Jen Mo—channel of function]." Thus in T'ai Chi Ch'uan the complete circulation is the same as in meditation. It is the Greater Heavenly Circulation formed by the Tu Mo and the Jen Mo.

There have been many books written about sex and meditation. A popular book in the United States is *The Tao of Love and Sex*,[13] which has an interesting foreword and postscript by Joseph Needham. The author of the book speaks of using deep breathing of the diaphragm to prolong sexual pleasure. However, the production, retention, and transformation of sperm into *ch'i* is not discussed. Without this whole process, the goal of meditation cannot be achieved.

The technique called Double Meditation, in which sex can be used as meditation, must be practiced consistently over a long period, preferably between husband and wife, in order to be effective. For details of this technique see Chapter 11, which states, "The ancient Tao of Loving masters considered love, food, and exercise the three columns supporting a man's life." We have mentioned the exercise of T'ai Ch'i Ch'uan, and the Tao of Love is the double meditation.

Chapter 10 of the *Tao te ching,* which we discussed in Chapter 1 of this book, has important points to make about both the techniques of meditation and T'ai Chi Ch'uan. Hundreds of Chinese and Western translators have written different versions without making the text clear. James Legge, one such translator, comments that even Ku Shu, third sage of the Confucian school, "was not able to explain it to the members satisfactorily."

Many scholars have only emphasized the mental aspect, especially Confucians, who did not have a complete knowledge of meditation and Chinese medicine. I have checked every original Chinese character in a comprehensive Chinese dictionary and medical books, and that chapter of the *Tao te ching* should be translated as follows:

Can you bring forth the spirit with the vital circulation (*ch'i*) uniting it with the body to be one and not separate?

The goal of Taoist Meditation is to cultivate the physical and spiritual together. Chuang Tzu refers to Kuang Cheng Tze telling Huang Ti, the Yellow Emperor: "Your spirit will keep your body, and the body will live long."[14]

Can you concentrate your vitality to become soft like a newborn baby: "soft" is related to T'ai Chi Ch'uan, and the newborn baby refers to the spiritual fetus.[15]

The character of T'ai Chi Ch'uan is soft and light. The bodies of the young are soft; the bodies of the old are stiff. One of the purposes of T'ai Chi Ch'uan is to rejuvenate.

Can you clean your mind and be left without blemishes?

This line refers to the Taoist meditation of having the body quiet and the mind peaceful, nurturing the spiritual fetus.

Can you love the people and govern the state without cleverness?

This line refers to the state as the whole body and the people as the organs within. See also the last paragraph of Chapter 57 of the *Tao te ching*.

The Gate of Heaven opens and closes. Can you be like the female?

The Heavenly Gate is in the crown of the head, from which the spiritual baby emerges.[16]

Can you become enlightened and reach everywhere without knowledge?

This system can be compared to our modern industrial system. First we must produce agricultural material, which is equivalent to *ching*. The next step is the development of manufactured commodities, which is *ch'i* or vitality. Then follows the distribution process, which is equivalent to the circulation and the transformation into *shen*. The last step is the selling of the commodity for money. This is the manifestation of *shu*, emptiness. The money flows back toward increased production and capital.

NOTES

1. James Legge, trans., *Chinese Classics*, vol. 1 (Hong Kong: Hong Kong University Press, 1960), p. 393.
2. Wilhelm, *I ching*, pp. 342–343.
3. Ibid., p. 49.
4. Ibid., p. 53.

5. See Needham, *Science and Civilization in China*, vol. 2, pp. 426–427.
6. See Lu K'uan Yu, *Taoist Yoga*, pp. 20–25.
7. People over eighty use a special method to perform meditation. Chang San-feng used a masturbatory technique. (See *Taoist Yoga*.)

9. Wilhelm, *I ching*, p. 318.
10. *Texts of Taoism Part I: The Writing of Chuang Tzu*, trans. James Legge, p. 164.
11. Ibid., p. 417.
12. Ibid., p. 419.
13. Joan Chang, *The Tao of Love and Sex* (New York: Dutton, 1977), p. 102.
14. *Texts of Taoism, Part I*, p. 299.
15. Cf. *Taoist Yoga*, p. 14.
16. Ibid.

CHAPTER THIRTEEN

PREVENTION AND CURE OF SICKNESS

From its beginning four thousand years ago, Chinese medicine has recognized the mental and physical aspects of disease. Traditionally, the mental state of the patient was considered to be even more important than the physical symptoms. Recently a new field of Western medical research, called psychoneuroimmunology, has emerged. Psychoneuroimmunology is the study of the effect of emotions on disease. As reported in the *New York Times,* "The new studies strongly indicate . . . that virtually every ill that can befall the body from the common cold to cancer and heart disease can be influenced, positively or negatively, by a person's mental state."[1] Today Western physicians and mental health professionals are increasingly recognizing the role of the mind in the prevention and cure of illness.

Meditation and Tai Chi Ch'uan are specific techniques for attaining peaceful mental states, which can help prevent and cure sickness. T'ai Chi Ch'uan integrates the body and mind, breathing and movement, hands and feet. The whole body becomes integrated and can move as one. The mind is used to direct the *ch'i* and to move the limbs of the body. The movement propels the blood throughout the system. This movement helps the functioning of the inner organs.

LUNGS

The open and closed movements of T'ai Chi Ch'uan are coordinated with breathing. This action resembles that of a bellows. The lungs are never at rest. Even in sleep, they continue to work. The deep breathing produced by T'ai Chi Ch'uan draws the breath down into the *tan-t'ien,* so that less pressure is put on the lungs, which thereby get a chance to rest. A famous T'ai Chi Ch'uan teacher had tuberculosis when he was young and began to cough up blood. He learned T'ai Chi Ch'uan and was not only cured but became a master.

HEART

Heart disease is extremely prevalent in the United States. It is the second most frequent cause of death. The deep breathing produced by T'ai Chi Ch'uan helps prevent and cure this illness. By using the mind to direct the movement of the limbs and to regulate breathing, *ch'i* is produced. The *ch'i* helps the blood circulate, which reduces the workload on the heart. Y. T. Liu, a friend of mine, contracted heart disease in his sixties. Neither Western nor Chinese doctors could help him. He studied T'ai Chi Ch'uan for one year, and at the end of that time his heart disease had been completely cured. He came to America and began to teach T'ai Chi Ch'uan. At the age of ninety-four, he is still teaching. T'ai Chi Ch'uan can not only prevent heart disease but also cure and rehabilitate the heart patient.

LIVER

The liver is as important to the body as the heart and the lungs. It secretes bile, changes sugar into glycogen, and affects the functioning of the immune system. If the liver ceases to function properly, serious illness can result. One of my students who suffered from liver disease had been tested seven times. Each time, a small piece of tissue was taken from his liver. Finally his doctor told him that his condition was hopeless. The patient then enrolled in my T'ai Chi Ch'uan class. At first his face was very red and he could hardly get up from his chair. Gradually he began to improve, and at the end of six months he was able to move freely. After one year he was cured.

KIDNEY

The ancient Taoists spoke of the kidneys as the source of life. If the kidneys are weak, the body is weak. If the kidneys are not functioning properly, one will always feel tired and be sexually impotent. In Taoist terminology the kidneys are referred to as the moon and water and the heart as the sun and fire. When water and fire unite, they produce great power. In the deep breathing produced by T'ai Chi Chu'an and meditation, concentration of the mind is directed toward the lower abdomen, the region of the kidneys. As a result of this warning of the lower abdomen, water and fire are combined. Another one of my students who had kidney disease was extremely weak. His wife had divorced him because he was sexually impotent. After studying T'ai Chi Ch'uan and meditation for a year, he regained his vigor and is now happily remarried and has two children.

T'ai Chi Ch'uan, through gentle internal and external movement, prevents sickness, strengthens the inner organs, and makes the mind peaceful. It is highly effective for specific medical conditions. For example, recently medical doctors have begun to advise patients with arthritis to move slowly and gently. If they move too quickly, they will worsen their condition. If they do not move at all, the arthritic condition will deteriorate, and they may lose complete use of their joints and ligaments. T'ai Chi Ch'uan would appear to be an ideal exercise for such patients.

The T'ai Chi Ch'uan movements should be balanced and centered. The classics say that if your spinal cord is correct and centered, the *ch'i* will reach the top of your head. In meditation the *ch'i* becomes spirit (*shen*) when it reaches the top of the head. In this way, equilibrium is maintained, and backaches and injury to the limbs can be avoided.

Nevertheless, many people suffer from leg injuries. Young people most often hurt their legs because they lose their balance or because they are overly tense. In older people, the bone marrow is dry, the ligaments are shortened and the joints are stiff. This leads to many leg and hip injuries. In most people, especially old people, the legs are usually cold. This means that circulation has not reached the feet. T'ai Chi Ch'uan and meditation direct the blood circulation to the feet, which not only warms them but also increases the bone marrow in the legs and prevents its exhaustion. The legs of a practitioner of T'ai Chi Ch'uan and meditation should always be warm. T'ai Chi Ch'uan is particularly effective in keeping the body relaxed and balanced so that one does not fall down. When middle-aged and older people fall down, it can be a serious injury which can bring on high blood pressure, stroke, or heart attack as well as broken bones. When people get older their bones are brittle or dry, their blood vessels become blocked, and their bodies are heavier and inflexible. The movements of T'ai Chi Ch'uan increase blood circulation and prevent stagnation. The quiet of meditation produces *ch'i*, which regenerates bone marrow.

The *Nei ching* says, "Movement grows fire. Fire means energy. Quiet grows water. Water means marrow." T'ai Chi Ch'uan is movement and energy; meditation is quiet and grows marrow. Together, the two practices can be very effective in the preventing and curing of illness.

MEDITATION

In China, Taoist meditation has been used to prevent and cure disease for centuries. In recent years, western medical doctors have begun to recognize the therapeutic value of meditation. Dr. Herbert Benson of the Harvard Medical School, in his book *The Relaxation Response,* says that meditation (which he calls "the Relaxation Response") "may be used as a new approach to aid in the treatment and perhaps prevention of diseases such as hypertension."[2] Based on scientific studies conducted by Dr. Benson and his colleagues, the regular practice of meditation techniques lowers blood pressure, slows down the rate of breathing, and generally relaxes the patient. This relaxation response allows the body to begin to cure itself. Dr. Benson states that "we need the Relaxation Response . . . because our world is changing at an ever-increasing pace. Society should sanction the time for the Relaxation Response."[3]

The Latin word *medicus* refers to that which cures or heals. Meditation is sometimes referred to as alchemy, which is considered the ancient forerunner of chemistry. We know that our bodies contain many chemical elements such as carbon, iron, zinc, and so forth. The inner organs in particular both contain and produce these elements. Each element has different functions—to repair or build up the cells, to produce oxygen, to flush toxins out of the bloodstream. According to Chinese medicine, there are five elements that represent five inner organs—fire = heart; wood = liver; metal = lung; earth = spleen, stomach; water = kidney. The theory of treatment of disease both in acupuncture and medicine is based on maintaining the proper balance between the five elements.

Meditation consists of using the mind to direct the breath so that all elements in the body are gathered up, heated, and transformed into an elixir. This elixir is called the golden pill or the golden flower by Taoists. In modern scientific terms, the elixir is actually sexual energy. The presence or absence of sexual energy is very important to the health and well-being of the body. When sexual energy is at a high level, the body will be healthy; when it is exhausted, the body will die.

Inner elixir can be produced by meditation and T'ai Chi Ch'uan. Both methods utilize correct forms and mind-directed breathing to cure ailments such as backache. This complaint is very prevalent today. According to one estimate as many as 7.5 million Americans suffer from backaches. In meditation and T'ai Chi Ch'uan, the back or spinal column is held erect, but not still, and is lubricated and strengthened.

Today, many news stories tell how harmful chemicals are causing serious illness and death. Many people have been relocated because of nuclear waste contamination near their homes. Fishing grounds have been poisoned by chemical by-products of industry. The Environmental Protection Agency has warned the public about dioxin. It has been found that many preservatives in food and seasonings served in restaurants are extremely dangerous. Once these poisons are in the system they can do great harm. Regular practice of T'ai Chi Ch'uan and meditation can help the body get rid of these harmful chemicals by neutralizing them, as it aids digestion.

Both T'ai Chi Ch'uan and meditation should be practiced daily. If you stop watering a flower, it will wither and dry up.

THE SIX SENTIMENTS

T'ai Chi Ch'uan and Meditation can also help prevent and cure mental suffering brought on by the six sentiments or emotions. These techniques can be used to cultivate humility and detachment. As the following stories of Chuang Tzu illustrate, the enlightened, indifferent attitude toward suffering frees one from it.

GRIEF

Hu'i Shih went to express condolences to Chuang Tzu on the death of his wife and found Chuang Tzu singing and beating on a basin. When questioned as to his sorrow regarding his wife's death, he replied that his wife was resting in the largest of abodes and to mourn her with much unhappiness would be not to understand Fate.[4]

People who have lost a close relative such as a spouse or child feel sadness; this sadness can easily lead to mental or physical illness. One of my friends lost his mind when his son died. The daughter of another friend committed suicide, and he himself subsequently developed cancer. There is no help for death. What is lost is lost. Chuang Tzu's reply to his friend about his wife's death is an example of the Taoist idea that life is a journey and death is returning home. Even Confucianists believe that death is natural, like the disciple of Confucius who quoted the ancient saying "Death and life have their destiny."

FEAR

> Two of Chuang Tzu's characters suddenly develop tumors on their elbows. When one asks the other if he dislikes the tumor he replies, "No. Why should I? Life itself is a loan. We borrow it and live. A living thing is but dust and dirt. Death and life are comparable to day and night, and while you and I were observing transformation, a transformation reached me. Why should I dislike it?"[5]

In this dialogue from Chuang Tzu's writing, the speaker is indifferent to his tumors and is not afraid to die. It is very important for a patient to be unafraid, regardless of the sickness. A peaceful mind can help the body heal itself naturally. The best medical doctors seek to console their patients—even when the illness is very serious, they reassure them and urge them not to worry. Psychology can often take the place of medicine. In China during World War II, medical supplies were scarce, and often there would be no painkillers for the badly wounded. It was discovered that if the soldiers were given a placebo of any kind, it would stop the pain.

DESIRE

> Chuang Tzu was fishing in the river P'u when two ambassadors from the land of Ch'u requested that he come to be a minister of state. Chuang Tzu, having no desire to be involved in the affairs of state, replied, "I hear that in Ch'u State there is a sacred tortoise shell whose wearer, the tortoise, died three

thousand years ago. And I hear the King who sent you keeps this shell in his ancestral temple in a sacred hamper covered with a sacred cloth. Was it better for the tortoise to die and to leave its shell to be honored? Or would it have been better for that tortoise to live and keep on dragging its tail through the mud?"[6]

Chuang Tzu was not interested in the high and powerful position offered to him by the king. Most people would think he was crazy not to accept such an honor. However, when someone is suddenly offered a high position, he (or she) becomes overexcited; once he has the position, there are many problems and pressures that keep him from being resourceful. If one day, he leaves the position, he becomes very sad. Many politicians who hold office become old and weak. Once they are out of office, they deteriorate physically and mentally and look twenty years older than they are.

Desire also includes craving for wealth or love. When people suddenly become rich or when they fall in love, they are happy and excited. But when they lose their money or the love of someone they care for, they become so devastated that they may lose their health or even their minds as well.

WORRY (TENSION)

When a drunk man falls from the cart he does not hurt himself as other men. Chuang Tzu says this is because "He knows nothing about the vehicle or the fall. Concern for life or death never enters his breast. Therefore, he is not afraid to collide with things."[7]

The drunk man in the story was relaxed. That is why he didn't hurt himself. Worry or tension should be avoided. According to Chuang Tzu, if you are free of worry, you are not afraid. This is different from taking precautions to keep from being injured or hurt.

A story is told in China of a boy who was home alone in the

countryside. His family was working away from the house, and the boy had made a fire to keep warm. All of a sudden the head of a wolf appeared between the two sides of the swinging doors of the house. The boy didn't know it was a wolf; he thought it was a dog. Grabbing one end of a burning stick from the fire, he thrust it straight at the wolf and said, "I'll burn you." Terrified, the wolf pulled back from the fire, and his neck became caught between the doors. The more he tried to retreat, the tighter his head was caught in the doors. Finally he began to howl in pain. The neighbors heard and quickly came to investigate. When they saw the body of the wolf stuck in the door, they killed him. The boy was safe.

The fearlessness and quick thinking of the boy had saved his life. Worry and tension, as shown by the wolf, cost him his life. T'ai Chi Ch'uan and meditation can help us develop calm, peacefulness, and clarity of mind.

ANGER

> Shih Ch'eng Ch'i went to visit the sage Lao Tzu. Arriving after a long journey he perceived that Lao Tzu was not a sage and insulted him. The next day he returned and retracted his insult. Lao Tzu replied, "Yesterday if you had called me an ox or a horse, I should have called myself an ox or a horse."

According to Western medicine, anger inflames your inner organs. It is damaging mentally and physically. A man once became so angry that he pounded fiercely on the top of a desk and subsequently went blind from the force of his pounding. When two people become angry they tend to want to fight and may injure or kill one another. The Christian belief states that if someone strikes you on the right cheek, turn your left cheek. Avoiding anger can prevent many external troubles as well as internal injuries. Everyone knows that the tortoises live a long time. They do not get angry or fight. Even if someone pulls at a tortoise's neck, it simply draws its head into its shell. On the other hand, boars like to fight and are easily angered.

They do not have a long life, and their meat is apt to contain toxic, cancer-causing substances.

HAPPINESS

Lao Tzu says: "The reveling of multitudes at the feast of Great Sacrifice, or on the terrace at carnival in the spring leaves me, alas, unmoved, alone, like a child that has never smiled."[8] This passage implies a concept of happiness very different from the Western idea. To the Taoist, indifference is happiness. Keeping your mind peaceful and the body rested can prevent overexcitement and fatigue. I've noticed that many people in the United States are very happy before they go on vacation, but when they return, they are often sick. This is especially true of people who go skiing. When they come back, they either have hurt their legs or have colds.

PSYCHOLOGICAL BENEFITS OF MEDITATION

Chuang Tzu and Lao Tzu were sages of the highest levels. Ordinary people cannot live like these men of wisdom. Their ideas, however, can be understood psychologically. Carl Jung, in describing the text of *The Secret of the Golden Flower,* the ancient Taoist treatise on meditation, wrote: "They not only lay far beyond everything known to 'academic' psychology but also overstepped the borders of medical, strictly personal, psychology."[9]

The American Psychiatric Association recognizes the therapeutic value of meditation. In 1977 it appointed a task force on meditation, which called the practice "a useful procedure in enhancing a sense of tranquility and sometimes alleviating stress and anxiety."[10] The task force also issued a warning describing the "disorganizational states during the practice of meditation which may be experienced by persons who are already disturbed." It is true that many people who practice meditation experience illusions that can lead to mental problems. This is because in many schools of meditation, too much emphasis is placed on spiritual ideas such as the belief in reincarnation. However, Taoist meditation balances the mental and physical in its transformation of sexual energy into breath or vitality and finally into spirit.

The practice of meditation must be carried out cautiously. The brother of one of my students was a serious practitioner of Indian meditation. He became mentally ill and was hospitalized. After his condition improved, he traveled to India, but had to be brought home and rehospitalized. He has remained in the hospital for the past twenty years. The former SALT Commissioner of China, Dr. Chu, was very diligent in his practice of meditation even though he was in his eighties. While meditating, he suffered from lack of oxygen and had to be lifted by two people and walked around before he could regain his breath. T'ai Chi Ch'uan and Taoist Meditation emphasize balance and proportion. One should practice slowly and proceed step by step, thus avoiding the possibility of physical or mental problems.

NOTES

1. *New York Times,* May 24, 1983, pp. C1, C8.
2. Herbert Benson, *The Relaxation Response.*
3. Ibid.
4. *Text of Taoism, Part II: The Writings of Chuang Tzu,* p. 4.
5. Ibid., p. 5.
6. Da Liu, *T'ai Chi Ch'uan and I Ching* (New York: Harper & Row, 1972), p. 8.
7. *Text of Taoism, Part II,* p. 13.
8. *Tao Te Ching,* trans. Ch'u Ta-Kao (New York: Samuel Weiser), p. 30.
9. *Secret of Golden Flower,* trans. Richard Wilhelm, commentary by C. G. Jung (New York: Harcourt Brace Jovanovich, 1962), p. xiii.
10. *American Journal of Psychiatry* 134 (June 1977): 720.

CHAPTER FOURTEEN

QUESTIONS AND ANSWERS

QUESTION: I have heard T'ai Chi Ch'uan described as an "internal exercise," while other arts, such as Shao Lin, are called "external" exercises. Would you explain the difference?

ANSWER: There are several reasons for the differentiation between internal and external exercises. Like Taoism and Confucianism, the philosophy of T'ai Chi Ch'uan originated in China. Shao Lin is the name of a Buddhist temple in the Honan province of China, but the founder of the exercise was the Indian monk Ta Mo. Like Shao Lin, T'ai Chi Ch'uan consists of many body movements. However, external exercises strive to build up the muscles and strengthen the limbs, while T'ai Chi Ch'uan movements use the mind to influence the breathing and blood circulation and to affect the vitality and spirit. T'ai Chi Ch'uan involves movements that help the inner organs, not just improve the physique. The practitioner attempts to develop a peaceful state of mind rather than a display that will invite applause and recognition from others. Confucius long ago observed, "In ancient times, people learned for themselves; nowadays, they learn for admiration." The goals of a healthy body and a peaceful mind achieved through T'ai Chi Ch'uan are directed to the abdomen. Together, the breathing, mind, and movement help achieve the goals of meditation—good health and longevity.

T'ai Chi Ch'uan should be performed in a quiet location and with a peaceful mind, like meditation. Doing these forms with genuine tranquillity, correct movement, and well-coordinated breathing (inhale, store breath, exhale) is more difficult than performing Sitting Meditation. But if all of these elements are combined correctly, the results from T'ai Chi Ch'uan are more expeditious than those of Sitting Meditation.

Q: How does one practice T'ai Chi Ch'uan as a form of moving meditation?

A: In the beginning, you should practice a few breathing exercises as a form of Meditative Standing. Later, you can combine several forms in movement practiced together. Start with the "inhale, store breath, exhale" form of Standing Meditation described earlier. As a second stage, practice the opening movements of T'ai Chi Ch'uan: Push Up, Pull Back, Press Forward, Push Forward. Beginning with Push Up, inhale as you initiate the motion, store the breath as the palms reach chin level, exhale as you Pull Back. In Press Forward, breathe in until the extended movement of the hand is 90 percent completed. Hold the breath. Then breathe out as the hands separate and your weight shifts back to the rear leg, "as if sitting." Push Forward again, inhaling until the movement is completed. All that is traditional like the practice of learning in ancient times. For these reasons, T'ai Chi Ch'uan is considered an "internal" exercise.

Q: When people practice T'ai Chi Ch'uan for a long period of time, they often belch and break wind. Someone told me this is good; someone else said it is not. Which of them is right?

A: When they happen and when they do not, both situations are good. The stomach and the intestines are "involuntary" organs: no amount of physical exercise alone can force them to move. But when the movements of T'ai Chi Ch'uan are performed correctly and the *ch'i* is directed by the mind to the abdomen, these organs may expand and constrict. Inhaling fresh air and exhaling the stale, you send cleansing blood and vitality to the vibrating organs. As a result, the digestion of food and the formation of wastes are expedited. Like the fumes from an automobile engine, gas is the by-product of the digestive process. Since burping and flatulence are means by which the body eliminates impurities, they are healthy and good, although not graceful when done in public.

A more advanced stage occurs when the movements are performed more skillfully and are more coordinated with the mind and breathing in the abdomen. Use the mind to sink the *ch'i* down into the *tan-t'ien* to avoid burping. Then use your mind to constrict the anal sphincter so that the passageway becomes closed, forestalling the escape of gas. The air can then be kept inside the body as a form of energy. This means that you have attained the meditative phenomenon.

Q: What is the proper method to hold the air in the *tan-t'ien*?

A: This method is called *shou-chiao. Shou* means "keep" or "store"; *chiao* means "cavity" or "center." Actually, there are many cavities in the body, such as the *ni-wan* (crown of the head), *mien-t'ang* (slightly above the center of the eyes), *t'an-chung* (solar plexus), and the *tan-t'ien*, below the navel.

Breathe through the nose. Inhale to about 70 or 80 percent capacity. Direct the *ch'i* with the mind to the abdomen, hold it there, then exhale. This general procedure is described in a previous chapter as a form of Meditative Standing. By doing it for a short period of time, you can store the energy. But when performed properly for longer periods, this breathing can create enough warmth to produce the elixir. You will be able to feel the elixir in the abdomen as a hard substance the size of a peanut or a little larger. In time, the elixir can move as a current of heat to other parts of your body. This vitality can cure or prevent many diseases and can contribute to longevity.

Q: Why do people call T'ai Chi Ch'uan "moving meditation"?

A: The form of T'ai Chi Ch'uan is like meditation. The body is erect, the mind is peaceful, and the *ch'i* and the perspiration are determined by our environment, our mental state, and our physical condition. The master sweats very little because his mind is peaceful, his body quiet and relaxed. Even the outside movements of the forms will not disrupt this inner calm, because the *ch'i*—not physical strength—propel his ligaments. This is considered a high level of T'ai Chi Ch'uan exercise.

Q: When I meditate, I always sweat—no matter what the room temperature or time of year. Sometimes I perspire very heavily. Is this good or not?

A: Meditation requires that you sit quietly. Even though the outside of the body is at rest, you will perspire when you are producing heat from the inside. In Taoist terminology, the heat produced by the *ch'i* in the *tan-t'ien* is called "fire."[1] To refine the sexual energy and the inner force of the *ch'i,* great amounts of heat are required. If the heat is not great enough, use the breathing like the "wind of a bellows" to intensify the fire and make sufficient heat to "melt iron." Melting the sexual essence to make vitality results in the creation of elixir.

Sweating is not harmful. Some schools of meditation recommend perspiring a great deal, for it is beneficial to the health of the body, expelling poisons, and is necessary to meditation. But before you meditate, you should protect yourself from drafts and chills. Make sure the room is clean. Open the window enough for gentle cross-ventilation but not enough to let a strong wind come in. Adjust the room temperature to not above seventy degrees nor below fifty degrees. After meditating, towel your body dry and wait awhile before going outside, to avoid catching a cold.

Q: It seems mysterious that breathing and the mind can make heat in the body during meditation. Can you explain this?

A: According to the study of human anatomy, the brain has two parts—one that receives messages from all over the body and another that directs the activity of the body. Thus, many emotions stimulate physical reactions. For example, if you feel guilt or anger, your body grows warmer; when afraid, your body trembles with cold. When ashamed, the face grows red; when frightened, it turns white.

Mental activity during meditation can create warmth in the body. The nerve fibers make an electrical charge when they are stimulated by the mind and the *ch'i*. It is this which causes heat. (See illustration.)

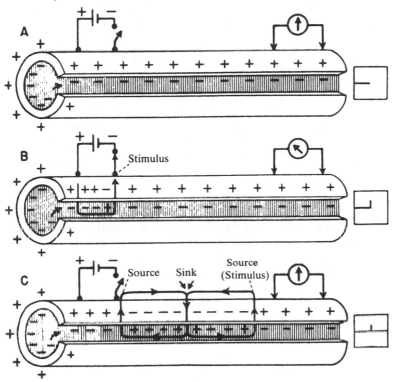

The Initial Change of Electrical Current in Nerve Fiber

Scientifically speaking, concentration, or sending one's idea to a certain spot, is to stimulate the nervous system in that region. According to modern neurology, nerve fibers are considered as hollow tubes, normally having a positive electrical charge on the outside and a negative charge on the inside surface. When a stimulus is applied, the charge is reversed in a small region.

SOURCE: Reprinted from *Creativity and Taoism* by Chang Chung-yuan. Copyright © 1963 by Chang Chung-yuan. Used by permission of The Julian Press, Inc.

Q: In meditation and T'ai Chi Ch'uan, the practitioner transmits energy through the spinal cord to the crown of the head. But this area is mostly bone. How does the vitality manage to reach the crown of the head?

A: As I have said, the vitality in the abdomen gets burning hot during the practice of meditation or T'ai Chi Ch'uan. This permits the sexual essence and other chemicals in the *tan-t'ien* to become *ch'i,* vitality. The mind brings this inner force through the body like electricity. When it reaches the coccyx, or base of the spine, the mind-driven vitality can enter a number of tiny openings that act as an entrance to the spinal column. The trip up the spinal cord takes many stages and requires much practice. Over a period of years, continued practice can make it possible to lead the *ch'i* up to and beyond each separate set of vertebrae. This will gradually pave the way for the vitality to reach its final destination, the crown of the head. This is a difficult task, but it can be done.

Q: If I want to do both meditation and T'ai Chi Ch'uan, which one should I do first?

A: It doesn't make much difference, but I can offer a suggestion based on my experience. In the morning, perform meditation first and T'ai Chi Ch'uan a short time later; you will then be ready to eat breakfast or leave for work. In the evening, let T'ai Chi Ch'uan precede meditation, after which you should be ready for sleep.

Q: When men practice T'ai Chi Ch'uan in the evening, they may later experience nocturnal emission. Why does this happen and how can it be controlled?

A: One cause of nocturnal emission is physical strain. If a man performs T'ai Chi Ch'uan too vigorously, the scrotum is stimulated and more sperm will be freed during sleep. In another instance, too much mental excitement during the exercise can cause nocturnal emission. Finally, some men who are overworked or suffer from exhaustion sleep too deeply to control themselves.

There are ways to avoid nocturnal emission after evening practice of T'ai Chi Ch'uan. Like meditation, the form should be done gently, with a peaceful mind and with a relaxed body. If the man is overtired, he should rest before performing the exercise or should only complete a limited number of the movements.

Q: At times, erotic thoughts disrupt my concentration during meditation or the practice of T'ai Chi Ch'uan. How can I avoid this distraction?

A: In the chapter on Sitting Meditation, I described the methods for keeping the mind free from thoughts. However, it is difficult for beginners to meditate or perform T'ai Chi Ch'uan without mental distractions. If, in meditation, a man's or woman's thoughts lead to sexual arousal, he or she can use quick breathing—exhaling through the mouth more than inhaling—to alleviate it.

Q: Some schools of Yoga permit sexual practice between men and women. However, I have heard that Taoist meditators restrict couples from participating in this activity together. Will you discuss this?

A: There are two schools of thought among Taoists on this issue. Taoist meditators do oppose sexual activity. They believe that it is best to accumulate and store the sperm within the body, and to purify the substance to become the inner force of the *ch'i*. In its purest form, the *ch'i* becomes spirit, which subsequently returns to nothing and then becomes sperm again. If this procedure is practiced again and again over a period of years, the sperm thickens into the elixir.

A second Taoist school contends that man and woman represent yin and yang. As such, it is claimed that the couple is indispensable to helping each other achieve the goals of meditation. As a defense of this view, Sun Pu Erh, the wife of Ma Tan Yang, composed the following lines:

It is necessary to have company on the journey to Peng-Tao:[2]

The single traveler cannot reach its summit by himself alone.
To think that the meditative path must be isolated
Is like crossing a river without a ferry.[3]

Both Ma Tan Yang and his wife used this method to help them
achieve immortality. The couple became known as two of the
Seven Enlightened Masters, and the government awarded her
an honor attesting to her state of perfection. However, it
should be noted that the method of meditation that permits
sexual play between husband and wife does not include con-
summation of the act between the partners. The man must
refrain from ejaculation so that the sperm returns to the brain
as a heightened form of energy.[4]

A branch of this school permits its followers to have children. Li Ch'ing Yuen, mentioned earlier as having lived 250
years, married fourteen times. At the age of ninety-six, General Yang-shen is a living example, for he has had dozens of
wives and has sired more than fifty children. However, it must
be acknowledged that special training is needed in order to
combine sexual activity with the more acceptable forms of
meditation.

Q: Many Taoist books make mention of enlightened Taoist
masters who have gone through life without eating any food.
How do they do it?

A: When the Taoist master attains the highest form of enlightenment, he has enough energy to live without eating and
without hunger. According to modern science, the atom is
very small but can release tremendous power. Nuclear subma-
rines, for example, run for a long time on atomic energy. By
analogy, the human body can run for long periods of time on
little or no organic food. Indeed, fasting makes the body
lighter and can lead to longevity and immortality.

Gerontologists say that older people die not just because of
disease but also because of the foods they eat. For example,
too much calcium from drinking whole milk hardens the blood
vessels of older adults. "Junk foods" are known to contribute

to sickness and aging. Eating fewer or none of these foodstuffs can make the body healthier and more youthful.

Many books mention the Taoists eating dates and seeds of the pine tree and herbs such as ginseng and others. Sun Pu Erh recommends a sparse diet of uncooked food and air:

> When full of the spirit from the nourishment of the air,
> You always feel comfortably cool and clean inside.
> You forget every circumstance, feel empty and light.
> Eat raw potato in the morning, magic mushroom at night:
> Cooked food will prevent you from becoming immortal.[5]

Swallow in the fresh air instead of food. Fresh air is believed to contain many good elements. Drink in the morning dew and the sun's rays[6] to abate your dependency on organic food. The proper method and conditions for swallowing the air have been described earlier.

Q: I have heard so much about Taoists becoming immortal. How do they achieve it?

A: Immortality is achieved according to numerous disciplines—including control of breath, temperature, and health. As mentioned before, we practice breathing to control breathing. A common cause of death is respiratory disease. Enlightened Buddhist and Taoist masters develop a great quiescence, refraining from breathing for several days. Another matter is the mastery of heat and cold. I previously described how the meditator gets warmth from inside the body: even sitting quietly, the practitioner develops perspiration. Conversely, we have observed, by the quiet practice of T'ai Chi Ch'uan, sweating can be averted. Masters who can control body temperature can wear the same clothes year round. In the 1920s I witnessed this in Beijing in the person of Wong Chin Tza, who wore linen clothing even during the winter. Taoists also use meditation and T'ai Chi Ch'uan to avoid disease and disability. Even though I myself have not reached enlightenment, I have stayed well. I have not spent a single day as a hospital patient, nor have I had any operations in my life.

At the highest degree of enlightenment, Taoist masters can even control the powers of life and death. They can live as long as they choose, and, if they want to die, they can cause their spirits to leave their bodies. Chao Pi Ch'en relates a personal anecdote to illustrate how the spirit can come out. He tells of his brother, the enlightened master Kuei I Tsu, whose body sat in a room while his spirit went out into the street and bought a cucumber.[7] For another example, Hui Meng (A.D. 638–713), the sixth and last Ch'an (Zen) Buddhist patriarch, lived during the T'ang dynasty. Today, his body resides in the Buddhist monastery Nan Wah in Guangtung (Canton) Province, where, although the spirit has gone, it has remained alive for a thousand years. As recently as 1976, the *World Journal* carried a story from Taipei of a monk who died eighty years ago but whose body still exists and whose hair and fingernails still grow.

Q: I know people who perform meditation and T'ai Chi Ch'uan, but I haven't seen anyone who has achieved longevity and immortality. Why is this so?

A: There is a Chinese saying: "As many people practice meditation and T'ai Chi Ch'uan as there are hairs on a cow, but those who attain enlightenment and immortality are as few as the cow's horns." In other words, out of millions of people, only one or two attain these goals.

To achieve enlightenment and immortality, four fundamental conditions must be present: knowledge, money, a guardian, and a quiet place to meditate. (1) You should get correct teaching from an enlightened master. Often, people who profess techniques of meditation and T'ai Chi Ch'uan lack these fundamental teachings themselves. How, then, can they provide you with the proper path to enlightenment? Rather than settle for "the blind leading the blind," take the time and effort to find a genuinely enlightened master. (2) Money is also important. If you want to achieve true enlightenment, you must practice meditation every day for many years. Therefore, you cannot distract yourself with the problems of making a living. You must be financially independent in order to make serious progress toward these goals. (3) A companion or guardian is necessary as well—someone to help you sustain your daily life by running errands, cooking meals, cleaning the house, and so on. When a meditator reaches the highest degree of enlightenment, the spirit can leave the body. At this time the guardian is especially important, for the body will be so deeply immersed in sleep that it will not appear alive.[8] The guardian must protect your body from all that might threaten it—drafts, changes in weather, even the danger of being buried. (4) Finally, the location of the meditation affects your ability to achieve enlightenment and immortality. For real success, find a place that is quiet and peaceful, similar to the conditions found at a Buddhist or Taoist monastery. The countryside may offer you the most accessible alternative, if the locale lacks noise and has an abundance of oxygen-giving vegetation. For further details on the benefits of a serene location, refer to the chapter on Sitting Meditation.

Q: Are these four conditions all that are necessary to achieve immortality? If so, surely the rich and the powerful— like the fabled Emperor Ch'in Shih Hwang Ti—could have become immortal quite easily. Why didn't they?

A: Emperor Ch'in Shih Hwang Ti was indeed a powerful ruler. Reigning from 246 B.C. to 212 B.C., he unified the territory of China and amassed great wealth. The Emperor employed many Taoists to find the elixir that would assure him of everlasting life, but to no avail. True, he possessed the four conditions I have mentioned—Taoist masters, money, guardians, and serene temples in which to meditate. But these are merely external conditions. He did not possess the essential internal condition of absolute tranquility and peace of mind, without thought, emotion, or appetite. Both Buddhists and Taoists say that one should eliminate the Six Sentiments— Love, Hate, Joviality, Anger, Joy, Grief—and replace them with non-thought, non-being, non-will. Therefore, Ch'in Shih Hwang Ti was too beset by ambition and the passions of power to achieve the inner peace necessary to becoming immortal.

The high officers of many dynasties quit their jobs and retreated from society to become immortal. A case in point is the military and political strategist Chang Liang. Around 200 B.C., he helped Liu Pang overthrow the Ch'in dynasty and become the first Emperor of the Han dynasty. Chang Liang refused to accept the prestigious post of Premier. Instead, he resigned from the government, went to the mountains, and, as a hermit, sought to become immortal.

NOTES

1. For further details, see Lu Ku'an Yu, *Taoist Yoga*, pp. 41–61.
2. Peng-tao is the mythological mountain of immortality.
3. *Book of Meditation for the Female,* Sun Pu Erh (Taiwan, in Chinese).
4. See Needham, *Science and Civilization in China*, pp. 146–152.
5. *Book of Meditation for the Female.*
6. Needham cites the practice of "wearing the sun's rays." *Science and Civilization in China*, p. 145.
7. Lu Ku'an Yu, *Taoist Yoga.*
8. For further details, see *Taoist Yoga*, pp. 160–173.

INDEX

About the Author

Master Da Liu was born in 1906 in Kiangsu Province, China. He began his study of T'ai Chi at the age of eighteen, under Master Sun Lu T'ang, founder of the Sun School and Director of the Provincial Martial Bureau in Kiangsu. During the Japanese occupation, Master Liu moved across China to Hunan Province where he took up the "softer" Yang style of T'ai Chi, under Master Li Li Giu, Director of the Martial Bureau in Hunan. As the focus of his studies became progressively spiritual, they led him to Ch'ing Cheng Mountain in Szechwan Province, a Taoist holy place where he met enlightened Taoists and T'ai Chi masters devoted to esoteric and curative work.

Master Da Liu came to the United States in 1956 and was hailed by *Newsweek* as one of the first T'ai Chi Ch'uan teachers in this country. He has written nine books on T'ai Chi Ch'uan, meditation, and Taoism, which have been translated into many languages, and has taught and lectured widely, at the United Nations, the China Institute in New York, and at Southern Methodist University in Houston, among other places. He currently holds classes at Teachers College at Columbia University in New York.